JUST DO THIS ONE THING:

A Guide to
Chronic Good Health

THOMAS MARTIN
www.OnePercentHealth.com

This publication contains the opinion and ideas of the author. It is intended to provide helpful and informative material on the subjects addressed in the publication. It is sold with the understanding the author publisher are not engaged in rendering medical, health, or any other kind of personal professional services in the book. The reader should consult his or her medical, health, or other competent professional before adopting any of the suggestions in this book or drawing inference from it.

The author and publisher specifically disclaim all responsibility for any liability, loss, or risk, personal or otherwise, which is incurred as a consequence, directly or indirectly, of the use and application of any of the contents of this book.

Wasteland Press

www.wastelandpress.net
Shelbyville, KY USA

Just Do This One Thing: A Guide to Chronic Good Health
by Thomas Martin

First Printing – April 2014
ISBN: 978-1-60047-960-1
www.OnePercentHealth.com
Cover Design by Brian Hirakami

Printed in the U.S.A.

0   1   2   3   4

For Elizabeth

"All truth passes through three stages.
First it is ridiculed.
Second it is violently opposed.
Third it is accepted as self-evident. "
                                        -Arthur Schopenhauer

Chronic: "persisting for a long time or constantly recurring"

SPECIAL THANKS

Without the contributions of the following people to my education, health and/or the editing, conceptual development, and creation of this book, it may not exist. Because I believe in its importance to the health and well-being of all people, I am enormously grateful for their expertise, input and belief in me and this work.

Elizabeth Fitzgerald
Anna Bement
Emily, Claire, Hillary &
Dorothy Fitzgerald
Mike, Dave, Chris, Peter &
Sam Bement
Robert & Peggy Sorenson
Ashley Wise
Susan Richardson
Kim Kornmaier
Sandy Coleman
Jonathan & Lyn Young
H.B. & Pam Wise
Barbara Katzka

Tim & Cara Grimwood
Marla Rothfisch
Dr. David Brownstein

Kelly Moeggenborg

Dr. Kevin Farrar
Dr. Lee Cowden
Dr. Dean Silver
Linda Ashton
Loraine Sorenson Martin
Cora Kveen Sorenson
Brian Hirakami
Roger & Kathy Massengale

TABLE OF CONTENTS

INTRODUCTION

"But I'm already healthy! I don't need to make all these changes in my life!" That's what I thought one month before I was diagnosed with heart failure (cardiomyopathy dilated idiopathic). I'm sure it was the same thing jogging guru Jim Fixx thought the day before he dropped dead on his morning run. I'm sure it is true of most people shortly before discovering they have life-threatening diseases. This is even true of people told by their doctors one week earlier, during a physical, that they are perfectly healthy.

But I wasn't healthy, I had heart failure. I was told I would need a heart transplant. I refused a transplant but I was dying so rapidly that emergency intervention was necessary. I had open heart surgery to implant a left ventricular assist device (LVAD). The LVAD bought me time, time to make decisions on what path I would take to find answers to my health issues. I have written about this in my prior book, *One Percent: My Journey Overcoming Heart Disease*. One percent was the odds I was given of turning my health and my heart around so the LVAD could be removed.

Growing up with a mother concerned about proper nutrition and from my own self-education on the subject, I knew I could follow the advice of the medical and pharmaceutical industries, which would lead only to a heart transplant, or I could take control of my own health. The body can heal itself as long as it is given what it needs to accomplish the task – this is the essence of holistic medicine. Western allopathic medicine primarily sees intervention by man-made, synthetic drugs leading to health. For the most part, doctors receive only 25 hours in nutrition in their schooling, so their view and the holistic view are usually in conflict.

Allopathic medicine has an excellent track record in trauma situations but a very poor track record with chronic illness.

Conversely, holistic medicine is not overly effective in most trauma cases but usually extremely effective for chronic illness. Before rejecting the holistic approach, I'd like you to think about yourself or a friend or family member with a problem such as dementia, Alzheimers, type 2 diabetes, skin diseases, or even cancer or heart disease. How effective has allopathic medicine been in reversing the symptoms or causes of these diseases? After an extensive study, Switzerland concluded that holistic/homeopathic medicine is more effective and cheaper than the allopathic approach. They now cover holistic doctors in their national health plan. [1]

Since my background is in software engineering, I took a logical step-by-step approach to my own illness. I researched the problem and sought solutions. Not everything worked for me, nor will it work for you. But this guide is intended to give you a starting point to reaching chronic good health. This book contains most of my daily and weekly routines and I am confident many of these things will work for you too.

When first diagnosed, I turned to a dear cousin of mine for advice. She has an amazing background in nutrition and holistic medicine. She quickly rattled off a list of changes to my diet. At the time, I thought, "This will never happen. I'm not going to do all of that!" But it did happen; I did make those changes; some changes I made quickly and others over a period of three years. I took them one step, one change at a time and somehow it all became manageable and possible.

So I did what was viewed as impossible. My heart healed and fifteen months after its implant, the LVAD was explanted.

I am back to life with my own heart and I am totally drug free.

Most importantly, if you think you are doing "everything right" yet are not getting the results you want, you might reconsider your health approach. To me, the only measure I have for right or wrong are the results. I reversed my heart failure and am able to live my life free of medical or mechanical intervention. I hope for you the same success by following the steps in this book.

The only time that hope is truly lost is when you give up or give into the disease. Cancer patients have been sent home to die by their doctors only to reverse the disease using holistic approaches.

In repairing my heart, I also sought the advice of several holistic doctors. In my initial conversation with Dr. Dean Silver in Arizona, I asked him how he happened to land on the holistic side of the fence. He said his story is similar to almost all holistic doctors; they all initially follow what they were told in medical school until they realize they aren't really curing anyone. And then, either they themselves get sick, or it is their spouse or their child, and they then realize they need to find real answers elsewhere. In Dr. Silver's case, he had a massive cancerous tumor on his lung. He was told by his oncologist to go home and prepare to die as nothing further could be done. Instead he sought the advice of Dr. Lee Cowden. That was over fifteen years ago and Dr. Silver is still alive and helping others today.

Although, I have written about my journey and discoveries in my prior book, *One Percent: My Journey Overcoming Heart Disease*, I discovered many people who have read my story and hear my revelations might agree with the basic premise, but they don't know what to do for themselves or, more frequently, they are overwhelmed by what I have done.

So I thought I should re-structure things so you can do what I was forced to do to survive: take one step at a time. I ask you to view this guide in a similar fashion. Make the changes one per week or one per month or even one per quarter, but start now. Some are very easy and some will be more difficult, but I did it, and so can you. In many cases, if you feel it is not possible for you to take the step and stick with it, just try it for three weeks (if possible). In many cases, you will see extraordinary benefits even in that short a period of a time. Hopefully, that time frame will be enough and it will make it easier for you to stick with the change. Each chapter can almost stand on its own: "Just Do This One Thing."

This book isn't about any one disease. Give your body what it needs to function properly and almost all diseases and ailments will heal. In fact, a healthy body is in a constant state of healing by removing dead cells and replacing them with healthy ones. Our bones are kept healthy by this same model, old dead bone cells are removed and replaced by new and healthy cells. One example of the problems with the allopathic model is osteoporosis drugs. These drugs stop the removal of the bad cells and allow only the addition of the new. By doing this we then place new healthy bone cells over old, dead cells. Yes, the bones will become thicker, but ultimately weaker. This was written about in mid-2000 by Dr. David Brownstein in his book *Drugs that Don't Work and Natural Therapies That Do!* He predicted we would see horrible bone fractures in patients taking these drugs. His prediction has come true and lawyers are now circling and suing the Big Pharmaceutical ("Big Pharma") companies for women sustaining horrific and sometimes unexplainable fractures, especially to their thigh bones and hips.

This book is about taking responsibility for your own health. With "Death by Medicine" being the third highest cause of death in the United States (by misdiagnosis, mistreatment and "acceptable" deaths from adverse drug reactions) it behooves all of us to be alert, aware and responsible.

The following data shows the dangers for patients in hospitals and is from the article *Death by Medicine* [2]

Type	Number of Deaths	Cost
Adverse Drug Reactions	106,000	$12 billion
Medical Error	98,000	$2 billion
Bedsores	115,000	$55 billion
Infection	88,000	$5 billion
Malnutrition	108,800	-
Outpatients	199,000	$77 billion
Unnecessary Procedures	37,136	$122 billion
Surgery-related	32,000	$9 billion
Total	**783,936**	**$282 billion**

The next time someone cautions you about taking a holistic approach over an allopathic approach to medicine, show them this chart.

I am amazed so many people believe answers to illness and wellness need to be complex to be true. Doubtlessly, if the symptoms of scurvy were to appear today (e.g. gums pulling away from teeth, loss of teeth, lethargy, shortness of breath, bone pain and eventually death) and people were told to simply drink lime, lemon or orange juice, they would protest. "That's too simple, too good to be true!" Provide your body with what it needs and it will heal itself.

This attitude is not new. While sitting in church one morning the Old Testament lesson came from Second Kings, the fifth chapter. Naaman suffered from leprosy and went to Israel at the suggestion of his slave, a young Israelite girl, to see Elijah. Elijah sent his own servant to meet Naaman and told him to dip himself into the river Jordan seven times. Naaman protested saying, "Are not [. . .] the rivers of Damascus better than all the water of Israel? Could I not wash in them and be clean?" Naaman's servant approached and said "Father, if the prophet had commanded you to do something difficult, would you not have done it?"

I see people resign themselves to chemotherapy, transplants, and even amputation while scoffing at dietary changes. I cannot understand why so many believe a simple solution cannot work especially since the traditional western allopathic approach is often at such a huge cost in both money and in long-term health. For example, cancer patients are more likely to die from cancer treatment than from cancer itself.

This Bible verse is also relevant to my experience in that Naaman was quite put out it was an Israeli slave who told him to seek out Elijah and then it wasn't Elijah who met with him but Elijah's servant. Simply because someone has a degree in a particular school of thought that doesn't mean another school of thought is invalid when spoken by someone who doesn't have the same degree. I am not a doctor nor a nutritionist, but then Bill Gates impacted the computer world, changing how we do business, write letters, and even write books yet he didn't even graduate from college. My experience coming so close to death, healing my heart and discovering alternative paths in health is my diploma.

Once a year, the heart support group to which I belong, has a round table meeting where each member briefly tells their heart story. I was appalled the first time as too many related how fifteen years prior they had a heart attack, followed by bypass surgery, stents, years of statin drugs and dietary changes only to face more angioplasties, more stents and in a few cases, even more surgeries a few years later. I couldn't help but think of the quote from Dr. Phil, "So, how's that working for you?"

We have carefully watched our cholesterol and followed the recommended low-fat, high grain diet for over fifty years. What is the result? Heart disease is still the number one killer of adults in the U.S. The medical industry (Doctors, AMA, Pharmaceuticals and the US Government) is unphased and continues to insist their approach is correct, pointing to obscure studies of 50 to 100 people instead of looking at the population as a whole. So, you can follow their advice and likely end up in an emergency room or you can look at the facts and take control of your own health.

Take the time to read and understand each chapter in this book. I encourage you to delve even further and read several of the books I reference to fully understand the need for these lifestyle changes. This isn't only for heart disease or heart failure. The source material points to studies and clinical experiences whereby following the advice in this book will likely reduce your risk of heart disease, cancer, type 2 diabetes, arthritis, a host of skin diseases, dementia and fibromyalgia. Isn't feeling good worth the effort?

There are basically four steps to attaining Chronic Good health.

- Give your body the most nutritionally dense food possible
- Prepare your body to properly and fully digest those foods
- Eliminate foods which cause inflammation
- Eliminate toxins which damage our bodies

One objective of this book is for you to eat a more nutritious and traditional diet. Watch out for words such as "all natural." Keep in mind that mercury, arsenic and lead are all "all natural." This doesn't mean they are good for you as each is a poison. "Organic" is another word to watch for carefully. Ideally, we do want all of our foods to be organic, but labeling is more of an art than an exact science and the buyer must be very wary. One well-known milk brand proudly labels itself as organic. But the milk is also "ultra-pasteurized" meaning any nutritional value has been killed by heat. The milk doesn't even need to be refrigerated. Look at the expiration date on some of these milk cartons, comparing them to others. Why do you think some spoil in less than two weeks and others can last up to two months?

Throughout this book I have listed products and resources as references. I do not own a stake in any of these items (save for my own website and books). I list them merely for convenience. These are the products, books and organizations I use and to which I belong.

The steps in this book are not listed in order of importance, merely by logical grouping. The first few steps I would recommend as particularly important for almost all Americans would be Step 23 (Take Magnesium Oil), Step 24 (Take Iodine), Step 2 (Eliminate Sugar) and any or all of the steps in *Part II: Gut Health*. Magnesium Oil and Iodine both dramatically reduce the risk of cancer and type 2 diabetes, even reversing the ailments. Both are applied topically and are easily added to your daily routine.

Try to give each step a chance for at least three weeks. If you are having problems with the step after that amount of time, you might want to stop. Some steps may cause detox or withdrawal symptoms, in other words, you are likely to feel worse before you feel better. This is perfectly normal and I am asking you to stick with it for three weeks to let your body complete the healing cycle.

This list (these steps) is by no means exhaustive. There are many more things I do and changes I have made to my life. I have selected these because they seem to have the greatest impact on our health. This is a place to start, not end.

Q & A

Since the publication of my book *One Percent* I have been asked two questions repeatedly, both in reviews of my book and when I speak to groups about my experiences and holistic health.

"What are your thoughts or what have you done after your experience with heart failure?"

My primary focus has been to ensure my heart doesn't "back slide." I have continued with my health regimen and continue broadening my knowledge of natural options to become part of the one percent of healthiest Americans and living a life of chronic good health. I have made more changes to my diet and my process for selecting foods. Not only do I not want to re-experience heart disease, I also want to avoid other serious ailments such as cancer. I decided to write this book as the question often comes up when I speak to groups. People ask me, "What should I do?" as it seems the perception of the first book is that it applies only to people with heart disease.

"How has this experience changed you?"

I have become much more interested and motivated to stay healthy and to stay out of hospitals and away from doctors. I have also found that I have little patience with people who complain of chronic illness but do nothing to help themselves. I also no longer fear death. To come so close on several occasions makes you accept it and at times embrace it. I realize it is merely another phase, another step and it is nothing to fear. I fear illness more than death.

One very interesting side note is that I am no longer afraid to speak in public. I had a terrible fear and would avoid speaking at all cost. Now I travel around talking to others about health without a second thought. I guess coming so close to death helps put fears into perspective.

One thing I want everyone to know is there is nothing extraordinary about me. I set aside my fears and dislikes and found ways to make everything in this book happen for me. I *KNOW* each of you can do the same and experience the same health benefits of this approach.

THERE ARE ALWAYS OPTIONS: THERE IS *ALWAYS* SOMETHING YOU CAN DO

The most important thing I want you to know, especially if you have some sort of chronic or even fatal illness is that there are always options, there is always something you can do. Your doctor, no matter how highly revered or regarded, does *not* know everything. He may not even be interested in knowing everything and his ego may prevent him from searching out alternative approaches, especially anything outside of the Big Pharmaceutical machine. So, it is your job to take control of your own path to health and wellness. The resources and information are available to you. The internet has made information readily available and many health professionals are speaking out and writing books of their clinical experience healing patients.

As I have read and continue to read about health, trying to optimize my own diet and life, I find exciting information about healing approaches to heart disease, cancer, type 2 diabetes, Parkinson's, Multiple Sclerosis, Crohn's Disease, irritable bowel syndrome (IBS) and even acne. These and a host more can be addressed and turned around. But if you think it will be a quick solution of merely taking another pill, you are wrong. Most require possible lifestyle changes.

After embarking on my path to wellness, I was initially surprised by the number of my friends trying to discourage me. "You have to understand, this is just what happens when you get older," "You need to listen to your doctors," "Didn't your mother have a heart problem?" They all wanted me to resign, give in and give up. I chose to ignore them. I'm asking you to ignore those people and those voices in your own head.

One Bible verse I turned to for comfort during my own health crisis was Romans 5:3-5:

More than that, we rejoice in our sufferings, knowing that suffering produces endurance and endurance produces character, and character produces hope, and hope does not disappoint us, because God's love has been poured into our hearts through the Holy Spirit which has been given to us.

I learned over time there was a reason Paul put those traits in that order. Before you can cling to hope, you must first have endurance and character. Hope is like a shining beacon which attracts moths and gnats, things which can distract you from your objectives. Only through endurance and character can you persevere. My hope was that I could find a path to healing my heart. But I also had to remind myself that my path was not my hope and my path may have to change to reach my goal. Also, do not fear hope. I have found it interesting the number of ill people who reject any new information, information contrary to what their doctor tells them by saying, "I don't want to hear this. Don't try to get my hopes up!"

There are other walls, walls of misinformation, often created by the very organizations which supposedly exist to help us and to ensure our continued health. There are answers to cancer, both prevention and reversal, but the information is attacked in an attempt to discredit it by the US Government, the American Medical Association and even the American Cancer Society.

Cancer is a $1 trillion a year business; and these industries are extremely resistant to that changing. Watch the excellent documentary, *Burzinski* to see how different groups do everything possible to suppress knowledge of effective treatments from the public. In a recent sci-fi thriller movie, *Elysium,* wealthy people from earth form a new society. When a poor individual becomes ill, the "hero" tries to get the patient to Elysium for treatment. The same thing happens in the United States right now.

The FDA keeps effective treatments away from the masses under the guise of "protecting" them, while the wealthy fly to countries which permit these non-allopathic approaches and are often healed. The Gerson Institute operates in Mexico as does Camelot Cancer Center. Camelot used to operate in Oklahoma but was shut down by the government, again to protect us. Both have outstanding track records for curing cancer and other ailments. This is one reason why you need to take control of your own health because no one else will be there to lead you down the path to wellness. Watch the documentaries *A Beautiful Truth* and *The Gerson Miracle* to learn more about these clinics and their approaches.

Now, I am in no way suggesting that every clinic outside of the US offering hope to cancer patients is legitimate. But, successful clinics do exist, ones which have been banned from the United States. There is a famous cancer doctor here in Texas with a tremendous track record reversing cancer and he has written books on the subject. He finally surrendered his medical license rather than be harassed by the government. He is now able to help and educate cancer patients freely without threat of arrest and being imprisoned.

The path to good health is simply giving your body what it needs to function properly and eliminating those things which impair its ability to perform as designed. It isn't any more complicated than that.

There are always options and there is always something you can do to make yourself healthier!

PART I:

Balancing Body Acid and Reducing Inflammation

"The Work of the Doctor will, in the future, be ever more that of an educator, and ever less that of a man who treats ailments"
- Lord Thomas Horder

"Medicine is not healthcare – food is healthcare. Medicine is sick care. Let's all get this straight for a change."
- Karen Pendergrass

Our diets are causing the pH balance of our bodies to be more acidic and less balanced. By pH balance, I am speaking of your body's overall acid/alkaline balance; at this point, I am not referring to the acid in your stomach. The typical method of measuring your body's pH balance is via a urine test. Cancer thrives in a high acid/high sugar environment. Acid also leads to inflammation in our bodies which then leads to heart disease, cancer, arthritis, type 2 diabetes and so forth. If you reduce the acid and the glucose spikes you will reduce the risk of these diseases. Glucose spikes are the sudden increase in blood glucose levels after eating something with sugar or carbohydrates. This is the high many people experience after eating chocolate or drinking a soda.

If you currently have any of the ailments I mention above, they can likely be reversed by following the steps in this section.

STEP 1: ELIMINATE SELF-DEFEATING ATTITUDES

This is rather self-explanatory. Don't keep telling yourself why you can't do something, find ways to make it happen. Do as many of these steps as possible. The more you do, the healthier you'll become.

If something seems especially difficult, try to think outside the box, how you could accomplish the same thing with possibly minor modifications. This was my thought when I finally decided to start juicing vegetables and fruit. I know sugar masks most bad flavors. But sugar is on the "banned" list of items for me to eat. So I thought about raw honey. What I found was I didn't need to use the honey either, the juice tasted fine on its own. But these are the types of things you may need to do when facing a wall you feel you can't climb.

The road to good health is not paved with good intentions. To quote my good friend Kim, it is paved with persistence and tenacity.

In my prior book, *One Percent: My Journey Overcoming Heart Disease* I wrote a chapter entitled "The Fatalists." This is a collection of self-defeating statements I heard over and over again often from well-meaning(?) friends and relatives. We hear these from doctors, the media and government and have accepted them as fact.

For instance, "We are living longer and that is why we are seeing more disease." Statistically, this is not true. If you factor out infant mortality and women dying during child birth, we are living the same length of time we were over 100 years ago. Sad, isn't it – with all of our so called medical advances, we have done little more than improve a child's chances of reaching the age of eighteen. Not that this isn't noble, but if you are over eighteen, little has been done to extend your life. Also, as I point out in *One Percent* if this statement were true, we should see the highest levels of disease in the societies which live the longest. Of course the opposite is true; they live the longest *because* they do not get these diseases.

One other myth that drives me crazy is the fatalistic attitude of "it's in my genes, there's nothing I can do." One hundred years ago only 1 person in 30 got heart disease. Now it is 1 in 3. If this disease truly were only an issue of genetics, it would then mean the only people procreating for the last 100 years were people with heart disease. It isn't that I don't believe there are diseases with genetic origin; I only believe this excuse is overused when effective treatments are actually available. Nor do I believe that even if you do truly have a genetic condition that many or all of the symptoms cannot be controlled merely through diet. I don't believe in the excuse "<shoulder shrug> There is nothing I can do!"

Stop giving yourself reasons why you can't be healthy and instead start doing things to reach chronic good health.

Be on watch for self-doubt, as what works for one person may not work the same for another. I struggled for years finding a natural solution to my high blood pressure. I tried many combinations of nutrients and minerals and none seemed to work. But after my prescribed blood pressure medication caused me to lose a molar, I knew I had to find answers quickly. I went back and reviewed everything I had read and finally found a combination of nutrients which quickly brought my blood pressure down to a safe level. I was discouraged many times, but I persisted and found answers.

I know one woman who looked for natural cures to her arthritis. Being unsuccessful she finally gave up on this path and turned to a surgeon for a hip replacement. Instead of continuing to pursue other natural paths to reach her goal, she gave up and decided it was simply "in her genes" and nothing could be done. I'm sure this attitude was fostered by her doctor, but I found it very sad since the same issues in our bodies that create arthritis, also cause heart disease and cancer.

If possible, take this journey with a friend. I know there have been many times when I have been motivated by someone getting ahead of me and my steps. They start fermenting vegetables and I think, "Hey, they are doing this, why haven't I started!" I then jump into the arena as well.

Daily meditation and prayer are also extremely helpful. It is no secret stress causes havoc in our bodies and easing that daily assault can provide tremendous health benefits as well as keeping focused on the goal of attaining optimal health.

Find ways to make these changes in your life. You will be healthier, happier and likely thinner.

There is far more you can do beyond this book, especially if you have a specific chronic illness. But I encourage you to start here, get moving, and get healthier. I read so many books during my journey to chronic good health and I encourage you to do the same. Don't wait, though, until you know everything. Start with these steps and reap the benefits of my experience and knowledge on this subject.

STEP 2: ELIMINATE SUGAR

One thing which kept coming up in book after book I read was the problem of inflammation in our bodies. There are definitely things one can do to ease inflammation, such as taking aspirin, but I wanted to understand the source. Inflammation seems to be the root cause behind heart disease, stroke, cancer, arthritis and many other chronic ailments.

Sugar is by far the biggest common enemy to our bodies and our health. Even worse, though, are chemical sugar substitutes such as Saccharine and aspartame. All must be eliminated and should be the first thing you consider changing in your life. If you are currently drinking "diet" anything and feel you can't stop cold turkey, first try switching to non-diet and, then, begin weaning yourself from it.

Sugar acts much like a drug in our bodies so we do experience a type of high and addiction. We can also experience withdrawal-type symptoms when we stop its intake.

Sugar causes your blood glucose to spike, much like a diabetic. Although these spikes are dealt with by our bodies with the release of insulin, the damage can still be seen in things such as the inflammation in our veins and arteries, which eventually lead to the buildup of plaque, which then can lead to heart attacks and stroke. Stop the glucose spikes, and you stop the inflammation which then stops the buildup of plaque. Once this happens, your body can begin reversing any existing plaque buildup, and your veins will once again be open and happy. This is getting to the root problem rather than merely trying to block your body's own mechanism for dealing with the inflammation. It has nothing to do with cholesterol; it is all about sugar and carbohydrates. In fact, some studies show that the higher your cholesterol, the longer you will live. [26]

I also realize the need for something sweet is very real. I did not drink sodas before being diagnosed with heart failure, but I still needed to find something to drink now and then to satisfy my sweet tooth. I live in Texas where sweet tea is king. So I made my own version to keep in the refrigerator. I have included my recipe in the back of this book.

If you must have something sweet, try using raw, organic honey. There are even beverages you can make at home to satisfy your initial craving for sweet when you stop drinking sodas and other high sugar drinks. My main resource to healthier foods and diet has been *Nourishing Traditions* by Sally Fallon. This book contains many recipes for naturally fermented beverages, which are sweet and can help transition you from a sugar-addicted to a sugar-free life.

Most importantly, eliminate anything made with high fructose corn syrup (HFCS). This is difficult because, like soy products, it tends to show up in almost every processed food. HFCS is mostly made with genetically modified (GMO) corn which has been shown to cause cancer in rats in a French study. The following chart shows how pervasiveness of HFCS (for reference, 237 grams is approximately 1 cup of sugar):

Item	Amount of Sugar in grams
5 tablespoons Ketchup 3 tablespoons vanilla whipped frosting	20
4 tablespoons fat-free Raspberry Pecan salad dressing 4 tablespoons Lite chocolate syrup	20
1 cup Lite Tomato & Basil Pasta Sauce 1/10th pkg Chocolate Fudge Cake Mix	18
1 bar Oats and Chocolate Chewy Bar ½ bar Milk Chocolate	10 to 11
8 ounces Tonic Water 7 ounces Fruit Punch	22

The average American consumes 47 pounds of cane sugar and 35 pounds of HFCS a year, according to the USDA.

A recent study by UCLA shows that diets high in fructose (such as HFCS) can damage your memory and learning abilities. In other words, too much HFCS makes you stupid. I think that explains a lot of things these days!

Sugar appears under many different names. When eliminating it from your diet, watch for these names on labels:

Sucrose	Maltose
Galactose	Dextrose
Lactose	Barley Malt
Sorghum Syrup	Carob Syrup
Refiner's Syrup	Corn Syrup Solids
Brown Rice Syrup	Maltodextrin

What about alternative sweeteners such as Stevia and Agave? I haven't spent much time researching these, although there is a lot of information on the Weston A. Price website (www.WestonAPrice.org). But I do know that, like cane sugar and all other processed food products, the more it is processed, the worse it is for you. The best approach is to avoid sweeteners of all kinds. Minimize them in your diet as opposed to seeking the ultimate alternative.

Avoid all artificial chemical sweeteners, many of them, like aspartame, are nothing more than poison to our bodies. Never use artificial sweeteners for cooking. High heat changes the chemical structure of the sweetener making it especially harmful. Try to use the most pure and natural form of any sweetener, such as raw honey. To read more about the dangers of artificial sweeteners, read the excellent article by Dr. Michael A. Smith saying they are merely FDA approved poisons. [27]

The following is a list of the most common chemical artificial sweeteners. Some of the names you may not recognize but should watch for when examining the labels of foods:

- Acesulfame Potassium
- Aspartame
- Neotame
- Saccharin

- Sorbitol
- Mannitol
- Sucralose
- Stevia (although from a natural source, stevia is often considered artificial because of the amount of processing it undergoes in most commercially available forms.)
- Xylitol

So how bad is aspartame? If you consume a lot of it (usually through diet soda), the poisoning may manifest itself in some of the following symptoms:

- Fibromyalgia
- Spasms
- Shooting Pain
- Cramps
- Vertigo
- Dizziness
- Headaches
- Tinnitus
- Joint Pain
- Unexplainable depression
- Anxiety Attacks
- Slurred Speech
- Blurred Vision
- Memory Loss
- Buzzing in Ears

Is aspartame really something you want to consume? [3]

To learn more about the dangers of artificial sweeteners, read this excellent article by Dr. Mercola: Artificial Sweeteners -- More Dangerous Than You Ever Imagined [4]

Raw Organic Honey and Pure Maple Syrup

Sugar is bad, but we still want to sweeten certain foods. The best substitute is raw, organic honey, especially from a local source. Raw honey should especially be added to your diet if you suffer from allergies. Local honey acts as a type of vaccine to your body, introducing the pollen in a safe and non-reactive way. When the pollen is in the air, you tend to have fewer physical problems if you eat <u>local</u> honey. Honey is easily absorbed by your stomach and avoids going further into your intestines. Raw honey also contains various enzymes which aid in digestion and are beneficial to health and healing.

Raw honey is often available in grocery stores, but you must carefully read the labels. Raw honey has not been pasteurized or filtered which removes or kills many of the healthful and essential enzymes in the honey.

Honey has another amazing quality – it never spoils, and scientists don't know why. It is one of nature's most amazing foods.

When using raw honey, be sure to only add it to items which are cooler than 118 degrees F (a high warm level, but not hot). Higher temperatures kill the essential enzymes and, with it, many of the health benefits of using honey.

Maple syrup (the <u>real</u> stuff, not Log Cabin or Mrs. Butterworth, which are merely flavored HFCS) is also a good sugar substitute. I rarely use it because I don't care for the maple flavor taste in most foods. Real maple syrup is available at many traditional grocery stores and also at specialty stores such as Trader Joe's and many healthful alternative grocery stores such as Sprouts.

I use one teaspoon of rapadura (a very raw, unbleached form of cane sugar) each morning in my cappuccino. It would be best if I did not use anything, but I also rationalize that everything else I'm doing compensates for this one daily sin.

If you *must* use sugar, try to use one that is in a very raw form such as rapadura. The brand I buy is Rapunzel, Organic Whole Cane Sugar, Unrefined and Unbleached. For some reason, the word "Rapadura" does not appear on the package, but that is what it is. It is available on the internet and from many healthier option markets such as Sprouts or Trader Joe's.

STEP 3: ELIMINATE BLACK PEPPER

Black pepper lowers your body's pH balance (to a more acid state) rather than raise it. I used to put ground black pepper in and on everything. So, this was difficult for me to give up. I do miss the taste it imparts, but I like the idea of being healthy even more. Plus this is a lot easier to give up than salt (which, as you read further, isn't necessary to give up at all!)

Try to buy whole black pepper berries and only grind what you need instead of using pre-ground pepper.

This is probably the least important step in this book. If you are on a special dietary program, monitoring your body's pH balance and it remains more acidic than you would like, you may want to take this step into consideration as well.

STEP 4: START A JUICING PROGRAM

For me, a juicing program was my most difficult step and the one on which I dragged my feet the longest. But as I kept reading about juicing and the obvious need for vegetables, especially raw vegetables, in our diet, I finally had to take this step. Cooking vegetables, even lightly steaming them, destroys essential nutrients and enzymes our bodies need. My problem is that I hate vegetables, especially those which are the most nutrient dense. It doesn't matter to me whether they are raw or cooked. The most nutrient-dense vegetables are kale, collards, bok choy, spinach, broccoli rabe, parsley and Napa Cabbage. Joel Fuhrman has an excellent chart, on his website, with vegetable nutrition ratings to which you can refer.[30] I worried about the taste of these vegetables and whether or not I would be able to get the juice down. I found, like almost every other step I delayed, it was really no big deal. It was easy to do, easy to modify my daily routine, and easy to drink.

I researched buying a juicer versus the Nutri-Bullet, a powerful blender which produces a smoothie-type drink. A juicer extracts all of the juice in vegetables while removing the solids. In a blender, the solids remain along with the liquid. I think if someone is fighting cancer, true juicing is the way to go. But, a good juicer is more expensive than many blenders, and since I was mainly doing this for general health, I went with the blender.

I make my smoothie with a mix of baby greens of kale, spinach, parsley and Swiss chard. To that I add some mix of carrots, celery, chia seeds, blackberries, blueberries, goji berries, pineapple, broccoli, apple, raw almonds, whey protein powder, and water. Make sure all vegetables and fruits are organic. Many grocery stores now carry organic vegetables, which should be labeled as such, but try shopping at your local farmer's market to get the freshest fruits and vegetables. It also supports local farmers.

I drink one of these a day. I try to drink it on an empty stomach for maximum benefit.

The main purpose of juicing is to get vegetable nutrition into your system. The fruits added are primarily for flavor, to make the vegetable juice more palatable. Go easy on the fruits and try to limit them to those which are nutrient dense (fruits such as blackberries, blueberries, goji berries, and pomegranate). Pineapple is very high in sugar and should generally be avoided, but it also is excellent at masking bad tastes in the vegetable juice. It is what I use regularly (but sparingly). Apples also work well at masking bad flavors. If you are diabetic, the less fruit in your smoothie or juice, the better. This isn't supposed to be a "treat" it is supposed to be for your health. In general, the vegetables make you more alkaline and the fruit juices more acid.

This drink provides a nutritional wallop and also helps raise your blood pH level toward an alkaline state, which reduces the risks of inflammation related diseases. If you suffer from gout, this is an excellent way to help reverse the problem. If you do suffer from gout, be sure to add extra celery to your smoothie or juice.

Vegetables and fruit that work especially well to make your body's pH level more alkaline and less acid are the following:

- Cucumbers
- Chia Seeds
- Flax Seeds
- Figs
- Sprouts
- Dates
- String Beans
- Kale
- Broccoli
- Cauliflower
- Root vegetables (carrots, turnips, radishes, beets)
- Avocados
- Swiss chard
- Turnip greens
- Wheatgrass
- Lemons
- Melons

Get a good and varied mix of these fruits and vegetables in their raw state, and you'll never need to worry about many ailments again.

A great documentary to watch to help motivate you to juice is *Fat, Sick and Nearly Dead.* The title may not convey this, but it is inspirational and one of the better documentaries out there. I don't agree with everything presented, but the primary points are excellent.

The health benefits are many, but one of the most interesting posts I've read was from a woman with Vitiligo (the condition whereby one loses their skin pigment). She said after juicing for a period of time, her pigment began returning.

Juicing may create a detox issue. In other words, you may feel worse before feeling better. The symptoms are often flu-like. In the wonderful documentary, *Fat Head* they show a fascinating animation on how your cells react when switching from nutrient poor foods to nutrient dense. You clearly see why you may initially feel worse when starting such a program as this. I suffered tremendously when I first started juicing. My solution was to help my body eliminate the toxins through coffee enemas.[31] Coffee enemas are discussed at length in the excellent documentary *A Beautiful Truth* which covers Gerson Therapy. It isn't for everyone, and be sure you understand the correct way to do this therapy before starting. Many web sites detail the procedure. Also, the more nutritious and nutrient dense foods you put into your body, the less you will crave the bad foods you don't need.

Don't delay starting a juicing program as I did. You'll be surprised how good it tastes and how much better you feel. If you are carrying around a few extra pounds, you may also find yourself losing weight without any additional effort.

STEP 5: TAKE LEMON JUICE DAILY

Every day, take an organic lemon, cut it in half and squeeze the juice into a glass of warm water and drink it. You can often find lemons which are labeled as organic in many traditional and specialty grocery stores or check your local farmer's market.

This is a deceptively powerful yet simple step. Lemon juice helps detoxify your liver and, surprisingly, it also helps raise your body's pH balance toward a more alkaline state.

The format and title of this book comes from this one step. The aunt of my cousin Elizabeth was diagnosed with a liver problem as well as a weight problem. Elizabeth told her to take lemon juice daily as well as eating two eggs lightly sautéed in butter each morning. Not only did her liver problem improve, she began losing weight. It sounded too good to be true, but it worked. She was then motivated to make more changes to her life and become even healthier.

Food Matters, the people behind several excellent documentaries, including *Food Matters* and *Hungry for Change* recently posted these sixteen reasons to drink warm lemon juice daily:

- Lemon is an excellent and rich source of vitamin C, an essential nutrient that protects the body against immune system deficiencies;
- Lemons contain pectin fiber which is very beneficial for colon health and also serves as a powerful antibacterial;
- It balances and maintains the pH levels in the body;
- Having warm lemon juice early in the morning helps flush out toxins;
- It aids digestion and encourages the production of bile;
- It is also a great source of citric acid, potassium, calcium, phosphorus and magnesium;
- It helps prevent the growth and multiplication of pathogenic bacteria that cause infections and diseases;
- It helps reduce pain and inflammation in joints and knees as it dissolves uric acid;

- It helps cure the common cold;
- The potassium content in lemon helps nourish brain and nerve cells;
- It strengthens the liver by providing energy to the liver enzymes when they are too diluted;
- It helps balance the calcium and oxygen levels in the liver. In case of a heart burn, taking a glass of concentrated lemon juice can give relief;
- It is of immense benefit to the skin and it prevents the formation of wrinkles and acne;
- It helps maintain the health of the eyes and helps fight against eye problems;
- Aids in the production of digestive juices;
- Lemon juice helps replenish body salts especially after a strenuous workout session.

Drinking lemon juice can also help dissolve kidney stones.

It is a very small, simple change but one with many healthful benefits. Again: if this were difficult, would you *then* consider it?

STEP 6: ELIMINATE SOY AND SOY BYPRODUCTS

This step may be more involved than you might first imagine. Soy and soy byproducts are in almost every processed food on the grocery store shelf. There is only one reason for this: soy is cheap.

The soy industry has done an excellent job portraying soy as a "health food." Nothing could be further from the truth. Soy is bad for us, very bad. In fact, it is an anti-nutrient; it actually pulls nutrition from our bodies. This is the reason soy milk is fortified with calcium. It is there to replace the calcium our body loses as it works to eliminate this "milk" from our systems. Soy also strips the body of Vitamin D, which is essential to building bones. Soy consumption contributes to osteoporosis.

First and foremost, all soy in the United States has been genetically modified by Monsanto (see Step 9). Our bodies don't even recognize it as food; it is seen as an alien invader.

Soy also contains an estrogen hormone look-alike. It can trick a woman's body into believing she is pregnant and can reduce the sperm count in men. It also reduces the sexual interest in both. If a couple is having problems conceiving, the first thing they should do is cut out all soy products in their diets. The second is to drink raw milk (See Step 18).

Contrary to popular belief, soy has not historically been a major part of the Chinese diet. It was used primarily as a rotation crop – grown and then plowed under to feed the soil. The only people who ate soy regularly were monks in their attempts to refrain from sex, the estrogen having its negative side effects.

Most Chinese only consume soy after it is fermented into tempeh, natto and tamari. The average Chinese today only consumes about 2 teaspoons of soy per day and the average Japanese, only 1 to 2 tablespoons and almost always as a condiment and not as a replacement for animal protein.

Soy is *not* a good source of protein. Soybeans are deficient in sulfur-containing amino acids methionine and cysteine. Modern processing damages the lysine in soy. Soy is also deficient in

Vitamin B-12 as the compound that resembles B-12 in soy cannot be used by the human body; in fact, soy foods cause the body to require more B-12.

Soy contains high levels of phytic acid and phytoestrogens both of which withdraw nutrients when processed by our bodies. Instead of giving our bodies nutrition, soy actually strips nutrition from them. Soy has been linked to multiple cancers, including endocrine, thyroid and breast cancers. It is also linked to hypothyroidism.

Soy is especially bad for growing children because the phytic acids can cause growth problems. Soy has been linked to autoimmune thyroid disease in children. Most frighteningly, infants fed soy formula ingest the equivalent of five (5) birth control pills daily.

Soy Formula is NOT safe for infants to drink.

Watch food labels for Soy Protein, Soy Lecithin and Soybean Oil. <u>You will be hard pressed to find any processed grocery store product not containing one of these</u>. Almost all packaged salad dressings are made with soybean oil. Mayonnaise is made from it as well. Make your own dressings using Extra Virgin Olive Oil or Coconut Oil. Or make a warm dressing using rendered fat from uncured bacon. Uncured bacon is labeled as such and is available at many markets including Trader Joe's. The dressing will taste wonderful and will be much better for you. (Yes, you read correctly – rendered bacon fat.)

Exceptions to this warning are <u>naturally fermented</u> soy sauce, miso and natto from soy grown in countries other than the United States. Natural fermentation breaks down the elements in soy which are harmful to our bodies. Naturally fermented soy products are expensive and difficult to find. I use a naturally fermented soy sauce which costs about five times the price of a bottle in the grocery store. You can also use Coconut Aminos which has a similar taste to soy sauce, but is made without soy.

To get the full low-down on soy and the references to support my claims above, please read the excellent book, *The Whole Soy Story* by Kaayla Daniel. Once you finish her book, you'll never eat anything containing soy again.

STEP 7: ELIMINATE CORN

Like soy, most corn in the American Diet has been genetically modified (GMO). High fructose corn syrup is made from GMO corn and should be eliminated. There is minimal nutritional value to all corn and it is high in sugar.

A great resource for the dangers of corn is the documentary *King Corn*. You will learn how this grain is in almost every processed food we Americans consume. Another resource is the book, *The Omnivores Dilemma* by Michael Pollan.

Eliminate all breakfast cereals, especially those made from corn. Packaged breakfast cereal has been heavily processed and has almost no nutritional value. They are so bad that when a test was run on rats, rats were given the option of eating cereal or eating the cereal box. The rats eating the cereal died before the rats eating the boxes. [39]

Now, don't start eating cereal boxes, just stop buying it all together! As an example of the prevalence of corn in our diets, McDonald's Chicken McNuggets are actually 56% corn.[40] If you serve them to you children along with a soda, they get corn with the chicken and the soda is made with HFCS. That's a lot of GMO food in a small, developing body.

What is important is should you choose to continue buying processed foods after reading this book, be sure to READ THE LABELS!! You will be surprised how often soy and corn and other GMOs and non-healthy ingredients are in the products we buy.

STEP 8: ELIMINATE WHEAT

First read the prior step about eliminating corn. The same is true for wheat-based cereals. Did you know eating Shredded Wheat will cause your blood glucose to spike higher than simply eating processed sugar?

The book you should read to learn about the dangers of wheat is *Wheat Belly* by Dr. William Davis. This book gives you the full picture on why eating wheat (even whole grain) is bad for you. Another excellent resource is *Grain Brain* by David Perlmutter, M.D.

This step was more difficult for me than I first realized since I rarely eat sandwiches, because this meant giving up pizza and hamburgers, two things I really enjoy. But, it was for a good cause and so – out they both went. There are ways to eat our favorite food and still minimize the negative aspects. With hamburgers, eliminate the bun. In-N-Out Burger chains do this if you order your burger "Protein Style." Other fast-food chains are beginning to follow suit with non-bread and gluten-free options. You can also make your own pizza at home with non-gluten breads, adding your own sauce and toppings. There are always ways around "bad foods."

You may go through some level of "detox" symptoms – headaches and other fever-type ailments. Don't give up; keep going. It is similar to withdrawals of a drug addict, because you are, in fact, addicted to wheat and the glucose spikes which come from it. Like drugs, wheat binds to the opiate receptors of the brain; it doesn't make us "high," but it does make us hungry. Wheat also has negative effects on our brain and its functions.

This step could as easily be in *Part II: Gut Health* because wheat appears to disrupt our stomach flora leading to many of the same auto-immune ailments. A recent *Wheat Belly* blog posting stated that wheat elimination can cause symptoms to recede or disappear caused by rheumatoid arthritis, lupus, psoriasis, Hashimoto's thyroiditis as well as other auto-immune ailments, all associated with a poor gut function.

The other day I was at a Korean-style spa and most of the customers that day were in fact Korean. I couldn't help but notice how nice everyone's skin appeared. It seemed regardless of the age of the men, their skin was smooth, unblemished and taut. I realized then that the Korean diet is high in fermented vegetables (which includes KimChi) and also almost completely devoid of wheat. For years the powers that be have been telling us that the sun ages our skin. The reality is that it is wheat, sugar and a poor functioning gut.

STEP 9: ELIMINATE GENETICALLY MODIFIED FOODS (GMOs)

Monsanto is the primary company behind genetically modified foods. They have been behind Agent Orange, Saccharine, aspartame, PCBs, growth hormone and Glyphsate, all which have been linked to cancer and other health problems. Now they keep introducing Roundup® Ready genetically modified seeds. These are new plants, foreign to our bodies and the environment, which are introduced into our food chain for the sole reason of being resistant to their Roundup® brand herbicide. Almost all soy, corn, and wheat have been genetically modified.

A study was conducted in France where rats were fed a diet of 33% GMO corn. The results are shocking. Each rat was covered with large cancerous tumors and died. Since all soy grown in the United States is GMO (as I said above on the step eliminating soy), it is in almost every processed food you eat. So, you won't fare much better than those rats if you don't stop eating them. Photos of these poor creatures are available on *Mother Earth News*. [5]

Not only did the rats suffer from cancer, it was also found they had liver and kidney failures. Fifty percent of the males and seventy percent of the female animals on the GMO diet succumbed to early death at an age equivalent to 40 to 50 human years.

It isn't only in the produce aisle of the market where GMOs can be found. Almost every processed food contains GMOs. Since most corn grown in the US has been genetically modified (and heavily sprayed with the herbicide Roundup®), anything fed this corn will yield less than optimal results. GMO corn meal is fed to cows, chickens and pigs. So, can you imagine the quality and nutrient density of their meat and eggs? In the documentary *King Corn* a cattle rancher is interviewed. He tells, once the cows are put on an exclusive diet of corn meal, they must be slaughtered before the 120th day. I talk more about this in *Part III: Nutritional Density.*

One statement I keep hearing is, "Well, everything in moderation, I guess." Yes, your body is pretty amazing at handling poisons and other invaders, but with the prevalence of

GMOs, you are getting them from too many sources each day. GMO corn in your beef, GMO soy in almost every other product, GMO wheat in your breads – so, if you are eating a standard American diet, you aren't getting GMOs in moderation, you are overwhelming your body with them.

To stay current on this topic, I recommend joining the Weston A. Price Foundation (www.WestonAPrice.org). They regularly post and e-mail information and also send out a quarterly magazine loaded with healthful tips and resources.

The following evidence about the dangers of GMOs is from a recent article published by Weston A. Price.

- Scientists at the Russian Academy of Sciences reported between 2005 and 2006 that female rats fed Roundup Ready-tolerant GM soy produced excessive numbers of severely stunted pups with more than half of the litter dying within three weeks, and the surviving pups completely sterile.
- From 2002 to 2005, scientists at the Universities of Urbino, Prugia and Pavia in Italy published reports indicating the GM soy affected cells in the pancreas, liver and testes of young mice.
- In 2004, Monsanto's secret research dossier showed that rats fed MON863 GM corn developed serious kidney and blood abnormalities.
- In 1998, Dr. Arpad Pasztai and colleagues formerly of the Towett Institute in Scotland reported damage in every organ system of young rats fed GM potatoes containing snowdrop lectin, including a stomach lining twice as thick as controls.
- The US Food and Drug Administration has data dating back to early 1990s showing that rats fed GM tomatoes with antisense gene to delay ripening had developed small holes in their stomachs.
- In 2002, Aventis company (later Bayer Cropscience) submitted data to UK regulators showing that chickens fed GM corn were twice as likely to die compared with controls.

- In 2012, researchers found that female rats fed Roundup Ready-tolerant GM corn developed large tumors and dysfunction of the pituitary gland; males also developed tumors and exhibited pathologies of the liver and kidney.

So, how do you identify GMOs? Monsanto and other food companies have successfully spent billions of dollars stopping legislation which would force the obvious labeling of GMO foods. But, there are still ways to check.

- Avoid any processed food containing corn, cottonseed, canola or soy
- Check the PLU codes on fruits and vegetables. Avoid any which start with the number "8" and try to buy only produce which starts with the number "9" which indicates it is organic.
- If something you buy contains sugar, be sure it specifically says "cane sugar" as most others are from GMO beets.
- As stated earlier, absolutely no chemical artificial sweeteners of any kind
- Questionable additives to food. Those such as xanathan gum, citric acid, maltodextrim, lactic acid, dextrose, caramel color, baking powder, malt syrup, modified food starch, mono and diglycerides, sorbitol, steric acid and triglycerides.
- Do not buy any dairy product that does not carry the label "No rBGH." rBGH is a growth hormone given to cattle.

A doctor in Tampa, Florida (video referenced below), took twenty of his patients, with a variety of ailments, all off GMO foods. The results were astounding. He saw rapid positive results with Crohn's disease, Metabolic Syndrome, diabetes, common weight problems, headaches and many others. [6]

No long-term human studies have ever supported GMO safety. Shockingly, the World Health Organization (WHO) only requires a mere 90 days of testing to claim that GMOs are safe. As far as I know, no one has ever died from smoking cigarettes within 90 days of starting, either.

36

But – our government says GMOs are all perfectly safe. Caveat Emptor!

STEP 10: GET AN ALKALIZED/IONIC WATER FILTRATION SYSTEM

As of this writing, this is the one step in this book which I have not yet taken, but not because I don't support it. It is primarily because of the cost. This is the most expensive step and I am currently looking for ways to make it possible. It has the highest priority on my own step list right now.

The system I recommend from my own research is the Kangen Water System from Enagic USA.

I refer you to their site and sales staff as to all of its benefits. But one of the principal benefits is, as stated above, the raising of your body's pH balance to a more alkaline state. There are cancer survivors who did no more than drink this water and watch their cancer disappear. Read the below referenced book for more information on this.

The government basically controls our water and what goes into it. In many areas, the poison "Sodium Fluoride" is being added to supposedly reduce the incidence of tooth decay (although, it has never been proven to do as much. Read more in *Part V: Toxins*). Now the government is considering adding statin drugs to our water. (My opposition to statins is clearly documented in my book *One Percent* but a more complete resource is *Statin Drug Side Effects and the Misguided War on Cholesterol* by Dr. Duane Graveline.)

Don't believe the naysayers that alkaline water is too good to be true or that this is merely water. It isn't.

For further information on cancer treatment and this system, I highly recommend the book, *Killing Cancer – Not People* by Robert G. Wright.

STEP 11: ELIMINATE VEGETABLE OILS

The reasons to eliminate vegetable oils are many. These oils include corn oil, cottonseed oil, canola oil, soybean oil, and on and on. They are almost all from GMO sources, and the oils are extracted under very high heat, making them rancid. They may smell fine, but they create inflammation in our bodies like a flame to dry kindling.

Consumption of vegetable oils also increases our appetites and causes us to gain weight. Just when you thought you were doing a really good thing by opting for the salad at lunch, you find out the dressing is working against you and making you even fatter.

Vegetable oils should NEVER be used for cooking. They break down at low temperatures and become carcinogenic.

Canola oil is one of the worse possible choices. Health problem associated with canola oil include cancer, Alzheimer's disease and type 2 diabetes. Interestingly, all three have been on the rise in the US since we switched from supposedly unhealthy animals fats, such as lard and suet, to "healthy" vegetable oils. [7]

So – what to use? The best options are extra virgin olive oil and coconut oil for salad dressings and coconut oil and animals fats for higher temperature cooking (See Step 12). The best fat for high temperature cooking is duck fat, which is available on the internet, usually in French gourmet sites. The second best fat to cook with is pork lard.

A great book to read on this subject is *Know Your Fats: The Complete Primer for Understanding the Nutrition of Fats, Oils and Cholesterol* by Mary Enig.

STEP 12: TAKE COCONUT OIL

Coconut oil should be a part of almost everyone's diet. It is a healthy saturated fat and remains stable at higher cooking heats. When frying or sautéing food, coconut oil should be used instead of butter or extra virgin olive oil.

Any reference within this book to coconut oil, I mean specifically and exclusively <u>organic, virgin coconut oil</u>.

The benefits of coconut oil are many, but probably the most amazing story I have read is from a man with ALS (Lou Gehrig's disease). He continued to decline and became disenchanted with his doctors, as he saw no change by taking the drugs they prescribed. He read repeatedly about the benefits of coconut oil and that a healthy person should take five teaspoons a day. He thought, "Well, I'm far from healthy, so I'll take ten!" Along with the coconut oil, he also took magnesium oil (Step 23). He said the symptoms started reversing almost immediately. [editor note: the original article said tablespoons, not teaspoons. I am assuming it was incorrect] [8]

A new book titled *Thoughts of Yesterday* by Catherine Frayne recounts Ms. Frayne giving her mother coconut oil after she had already been deteriorating from Alzheimer's disease. The coconut oil smoothed out many of the rough spots, made her mother less combative, her mood improved and she conversed more lucidly.

Another story tells of an elderly woman distressed as she watched her husband slipping into dementia. She began adding coconut oil to his morning oatmeal. His mind became clearer and sharper and within a few months he was his old self again.

A recent British study shows that taking daily coconut oil can reverse Alzheimer's disease.

Coconut oil has been shown to help aspergers, autism, Parkinson's, ALS, dementia and MS. [9] In the referenced article, please note the clock drawn by an Alzheimer's patient before treatment and then two to five weeks into the coconut oil treatment.

So what are other reasons to take and use coconut oil?:

- Our bodies can rapidly metabolize the fats in coconut oil into fuel for the brain and for muscle function rather than it being stored in our bodies as fat.
- Eating coconut oil can also help control weight. A study conducted in 2009 found that women consuming coconut oil had greater weight loss in their abdominal region. The oil helps protect the body from insulin resistance. This lowers your risk of type 2 diabetes, heart disease and cancer.
- Coconut oil helps with digestive problems such as irritable bowel syndrome. The fatty acids in coconut oil have anti-microbial properties which have a soothing effect on bacteria, candida and parasites, which can cause poor digestion.
- It also has antifungal, antibacterial and antiviral properties which boost the immune system, protecting against h. pylori (the bacteria which causes ulcers), candida, influenza and herpes.
- Coconut oil can also boost a person's metabolism helping them lose weight and resist gaining more weight.
- It is also good for your skin when used topically as a moisturizer.
- It is also extremely good for oil pulling in your mouth, removing toxins from your teeth and gums. Upon rising in the morning, first thing, place about 2 teaspoons of the oil in your mouth and swish it around for 10 to 20 minutes. Do NOT swallow the oil, spit it out. This will help repair and reduce both gum and teeth problems, including cavities. [35]

I found a website challenging the claims of the benefits of coconut oil. As I read through the comments I couldn't help but wonder: "So how effectively is your doctor helping you? Has your doctor reversed the dementia or Alzheimer's disease in you or your loved one?" I already know they haven't, so why wouldn't you try coconut oil? Again, if it were difficult, would you *then* try? And what would be the down side of taking coconut oil? There is none.

I am constantly amazed at the resistance to trying alternate therapies.

I have struggled for ways to take coconut oil and finally came upon the best solution for me. I gently warm water and pour over the solid coconut oil in a glass. To that I add either freshly squeezed lemon juice or even a small amount of raw apple cider vinegar.

When taking coconut oil, build up the amount you take slowly. Taking too much at first can cause very loose bowels. In fact, this is an excellent natural laxative. Start with only one teaspoon of the oil and add one teaspoon a week until you reach five. If you have a serious neurological problem such as ALS (Lou Gehrig's disease), MS, Alzheimer's, or Osteoarthritis you might want to work up to even higher levels.

STEP 13: STOP USING MICROWAVE OVENS TO COOK, HEAT OR DEFROST FOOD

Microwave ovens help ensure you get no nutrition from your food. They kill off most enzymes and nutrients. People who regularly use microwaves have bodies which are starved for nutrition and their body pH levels are quite acidic. Add some sugary soda to this and it becomes a perfect storm for cancer to thrive.

Doctor Joseph Mercola has an excellent article on the negative effects of microwave ovens. [10] The following are several of his points:

. . . Microwave ovens in fact will threaten your health by violently ripping the molecules in your food apart, rendering some nutrients inert, at best, and carcinogenic at its worst.

Microwaves heat food by causing the water molecules in it to resonate at very high frequencies and eventually turn to steam which heats your food. While this can rapidly heat your food, what most people fail to realize is that it also causes a change in your food's chemical structure.

Another problem with microwave ovens is that carcinogenic toxins can leach out of your plastic and paper containers/covers and into your food.

The January/February 1990 issue of *Nutrition Action Newsletter* reported the leakage of numerous toxic chemicals from the packaging of common microwavable foods, including pizzas, chips and popcorn. Chemicals included polyethylene terpthalate (PET), benzene, toluene, and xylene. Microwaving fatty foods in plastic containers leads to the release of dioxins (known carcinogens) and other toxins into your food.

The *Powerwatch* article cited above also summarizes the Russian research quite well, which I will duplicate below.

- Russian investigators found that carcinogens were formed from the microwaving of nearly all foods tested.
- The microwaving of milk and grains converted some of the amino acids into carcinogenic substances.

- Microwaving prepared meats caused the formation of the cancer-causing agents d-Nitrosodienthanolamines.
- Thawing frozen fruits by microwave converted their glucoside and galactoside fractions into carcinogenic substances.
- Extremely short exposure of raw, cooked or frozen vegetables converted their plant alkaloids into carcinogens.
- Carcinogenic free radicals were formed in microwaved plants – especially root vegetables.
- Structural degradation leading to decreased food value was found to be 60 to 90 percent overall for all foods tested, with significant decreases in bioavailability of B complex vitamins, vitamins C and E, essential minerals, and lipotropics (substances that prevent abnormal accumulation of fat).

I might add this finding is supported by the 1998 Japanese study by Watanabe about vitamin B-12 in milk, cited above.

PART II

Gut Health

*"You can't keep one disease and heal two others –
when the body heals, it heals everything."*
                                             -Charlotte Gerson

In many ways, *Part II* could be the entire subject for *Just Do This One Thing*. The more I read, the more I find that optimal physical health cannot be achieved without first attaining optimal gut health.

A properly functioning gut is absolutely essential for good health. But the standard American diet makes this nearly impossible. We eat almost nothing which feeds the necessary flora in our stomachs and intestinal tract. In fact, we eat foods covered in herbicides (primarily Monsanto's Roundup®) which, although they may be safe to us as humans they kill the vital flora our bodies need to properly digest food and extract its essential nutrients. The EPA (you know, that Federal Agency which is supposed to protect us) increased the "safe" amount of Roundup® for us to consume in a year from 2 ounces in 2012 to 60 ounces in 2013. Sorry, I really don't feel "safe." [11]

Most skin ailments originate from a poorly functioning gut. Improperly digested foods become toxins to our bodies, which our body then tries to eliminate through our skin. These ailments, such as eczema, psoriasis, acne, acne rosacea, and hives, can be reversed by giving our system what it needs to function correctly, as nature intended.

The ten-year-old son of a friend of mine suffered terribly from eczema. It became so bad he was barely able to wear clothing. After a couple of years and many doctors and unsuccessful treatments, my friend sought the advice of a holistic doctor near him. The doctor put him on a battery of probiotic capsules, and the eczema began to subside almost immediately.

Other ailments associated with low stomach acid and poor flora are allergies, leaky gut and autoimmune disorders such as Hashimoto's disease, Graves' disease, Lupus and rheumatoid and psoriatic arthritis, migraine headaches and even persistently bad breath.

If following the steps in this book are not enough to reverse your problem, you may want to take the next step and start what is called the GAPS (Gut and Psychology) or SCD (Specific Carbohydrate Diet) Diets. To delve into this further, read, *Breaking the Vicious Cycle* by Elaine Gloria Gottschall.

Other diseases which can be positively affected by a properly functioning gut are diabetes, heart disease and respiratory infections (common with colds and the flu), asthma, and cancer (especially colon cancer). A posting on my blog [32] goes into far more detail about the positive effects on the body by improving gut health.

Amazingly, good gut health has even been shown to reverse many of the symptoms of autism. This has especially been shown through autistic children on the GAPS diet. Good gut health can also reverse the negative symptoms of ADD/ADHD.

The following steps are critical to good health. What is interesting is that, once your gut works properly, you may find yourself losing weight without changing anything else in your diet. One documentary I watched, told of a very obese man who first tackled weight loss through gut health. In one day, he lost over 10 pounds, through bowel movements alone. My entire life I had only one bowel movement a day, first thing in the morning. I remember a naturopath telling me that if I ate three meals a day, I should also have three bowel movements a day. I thought, how is that supposed to happen; by taking laxatives? Certainly that couldn't be the solution?

Once I started taking my gut health seriously, many things started to change; most noticeably, I went from one to three to four bowel movements a day, and I felt much better in general.

Women should think about how much they spend on skin products. The answer may not be in a jar, but in your kitchen by which foods you eat and avoid.

STEP 14: MAKE YOUR OWN YOGURT

Yogurt provides some of the flora your stomach needs to properly process and digest food.

This was another step in which I foolishly dragged my feet for a long while. I have eaten and loved yogurt since I was a teenager. What I later found was that I loved all of the sugar and high fructose corn syrup in most of the yogurt brands on the shelf. On a trip to France in 2000, I had pure, unflavored yogurt in a small glass jar. As I ate the luscious cream, I thought, "Oh, so this is what yogurt *really* tastes like!"

I stopped eating grocery store yogurt when I returned to the U.S. I started eating Strauss yogurt, plain and whole fat (which is the only form anyone should eat – never low fat or low calorie). The only ingredients besides milk that should be on the label of the yogurt you buy (if you won't make your own) should be culture and *possibly* gelatin.

When I lost my source for Strauss yogurt, I knew it was time for me to take the next step and make my own. Based on the recommendation of my cousin, I bought a YoGourmet Yogurt maker. It is available from many sources including Amazon. I also buy their brand of dehydrated culture mix.

It didn't take long before it simply became part of my weekly routine. I use a new packet of culture mix with each batch. I also use raw, whole milk when making the yogurt. (You can read more about raw milk in Step 18). If you do not have access to raw milk, instead try to find non-homogenized milk, often called "Cream Top."

Instead of using a new packet of culture with each batch, you *can* take a small amount of yogurt from an earlier batch and incorporate it into the new. The downside of this is that each subsequent batch will have less and less culture, the part of yogurt especially beneficial to our bodies.

It you want to flavor your yogurt, my favorite combination is fresh lemon juice and a drizzle of raw, organic honey. It's good and good for you.

Store bought yogurt is unlikely to contain a sufficient amount of healthful, gut bacteria, so it is very beneficial to make your own. The wonderful taste of the yogurt and the health benefits are worth it.

Perhaps you can also find creative ways to consume yogurt. I suggest putting it into a smoothie with fresh fruit (especially super fruits such as blueberries, goji berries, and blackberries).

If you absolutely cannot make yogurt, I suggest checking the Weston A. Price Shopping Guide for the top brands they recommend that you can find in your market.

For more information on the benefits of eating yogurt, read the following article on my own website. [12]

This is an important and delicious step. Don't hesitate to start.

STEP 15: FERMENT YOUR OWN VEGETABLES

No step has had as great an impact on me as when I started fermenting and eating my own vegetables. This was another step I delayed far too long and one so simple that I can't understand why I was so hesitant to start.

The two most important vegetables to start your fermentation lifestyle are cabbage and celery. Both contain a lot of moisture. To these I usually add ginger, carrots, garlic, daikon radish and often other root vegetables.

I read several recipes and watched many do-it-yourself (DIY) videos to produce my basic recipe which is included at the end of this book. Another great resource is the book *Fermented* by Jill Ciciarelli. Look for my own videos on YouTube on making both yogurt and fermented vegetables. There will be a link to it on my own website: www.OnePercentHealth.com.

I try to eat a large spoonful every day, sometimes by itself and sometimes putting it atop other foods. This gets my gut working like a champ! If you don't have time to eat some of the vegetables, at least take a small amount of the liquid and drink it. You'll still get the beneficial bacteria your gut so desperately needs.

If you can't take the time to ferment your own vegetables, try to buy them from the store. Be sure they are actually fermented versus merely "pickled." One great brand to buy is Bubbies. Their sauerkraut is excellent.

STEP 16: DRINK KOMBUCHA/KVASS/ KEFIR/TAKE PROBIOTIC CAPSULES

Proper gut health requires the ingestion of cultures and bacteria necessary for it to function as intended, both breaking down food and properly absorbing the nutrition within. Kombucha tea is a wonder drink. It can be brewed at home or purchased from many health food stores, under brand names such as *Synergy*. Many look like fruit drinks, but be aware that they taste more like mild wine and can be a bit sour. They will also be lightly effervescent.

Consumed regularly, kombucha can help you lose excess water weight, swelling and fluid which accumulate in your tissues from alcohol and processed foods high in chemicals.

Kombucha helps with detoxification of the liver, which aides in cancer prevention and reversal. It is rich in enzymes and bacterial acids that your body needs to naturally detoxify, thus reducing the load on your pancreas. Kombucha is very high in glucaric acid, which helps prevent cancer. Kombucha also contains glucosamines which prevent and treat all forms of arthritis.

With 70% of your immune system in your gut, the probiotic cultures and enzymes in kombucha make you more resistant to cold, flu and infections.

Kvass is another excellent beverage made from black or regular rye bread or from beets. Like Kombucha, it provides a wonderful hit of probiotics to our digestive system. Refer to *Nourishing Traditions* by Sally Fallon for recipes for a variety of fermented drinks, including Kvass.

You may also purchase and take probiotics capsules such as Bio-Kult. But, like almost any healthy food, it is best to get probiotics naturally.

STEP 17: TAKE BETAINE HCL TABLETS

If you suffer from chronic heartburn or acid reflux – unlike what we have been told for years – the problem isn't too much acid, it is too little acid compared to the amount of food you are eating.[33] Our bodies need hydrochloric acid in our stomachs to digest food. How then can introducing a tablet to neutralize that acid be helpful? The answer, of course, is it isn't. It is a trick to get our body to produce more acid. We take the antacid, it neutralizes the stomach acid so a message goes to our brain saying, "What's going on here? There is no acid in the stomach!" Our bodies then dump more acid into the stomach and the food is properly broken down.

Do not confuse the acid in your stomach with your body's overall pH acid/alkaline balance.

Asthma patients generally have low to no hydrochloric acid production. Eighty years ago a physician placed asthmatic children on HCL therapy (having these children take Betaine HCL tablets.) and noticed that most symptoms significantly improved. This along with eliminating processed foods and switching to a nutrient dense diet and increasing gut flora will give great relief to the sufferers of asthma.

I had a life-long problem with stomach gas that started a vicious cycle of hiccups which could go on for days. I finally found that an over-the-counter brand of tablets could break apart the gas and stop the hiccups. The problem was I would have to take many of them – more than recommended – and I would feel physically terrible after. Now I take two or three Betaine HCL tablets and, within an hour, the problem is gone.

I also found as I aged that I had problems in the middle of the night with acid reflux. I would awaken with the sensation I needed to vomit with acid moving up my esophagus. Now, when this happens, I immediately rise, take two or three tablets with water, wait a short while and return to bed. The problem is gone. The better approach, when I remember, is to take the tablets immediately after dinner, especially if the dinner is unusually large or late in the evening.

One major antacid product once claimed in their commercials that they are made with calcium and it is something your body needs. The latter is true, but the calcium in their product is calcium carbonate – not only the cheapest form of calcium, but one that neutralizes acid, thus preventing your body from absorbing the calcium. If you take calcium supplements, be sure to take Calcium Citrate as well as magnesium (preferably magnesium oil (see Step 23)), vitamin D3 and vitamin K2 for proper absorption.

Listen or read the warnings on drugs available to eliminate acid reflux. They include low magnesium levels. This would then lead to poor calcium absorption and ultimately osteoporosis. Does this really sound like a product you want to take?

A great read on this topic is *Why Stomach Acid Is Good For You: Natural Relief from Heartburn, Indigestion, Reflux and GERD* by Jonathan Wright.

PART III

Nutritional Density

"We are poisoning ourselves with highly processed, nutrient deficient food."

-Dr. Ian Brighthope

"The key to eating healthy? Avoid any food that has a TV commercial."

-Dr. Julian Whitaker

"What would happen if everybody ate lots and lots of fresh organic food that was minimally processed? I think we'd have an epidemic of health."

-Dr. Andrew Saul

I keep hearing the medical community say we get all the nutrition we need from food. That is the ideal and truly is the best way to get nutrition, but foods available in most stores and restaurants (especially fast food) are almost completely devoid of any nutrition. This is especially true of food cooked in microwave ovens. (See Step 13). You must seek nutrient-dense foods, i.e. foods which contain the highest levels of nutrition, vitamins, minerals and enzymes that are needed by your body to function at optimal levels of health.

Even fruit and vegetables in the produce section of your markets may be modified or treated for "shelf life" rather than nutrition. A recent study took grocery store oranges and tested them. They were found to be without any vitamin C. But, they sure do look pretty on the shelf! Oranges are also often dyed orange, again to look good on the shelf. Sad, isn't it.

If you want to be healthy, you must provide your body with the best possible foods, and those foods are the ones which are nutrient dense. Your body will come alive when given what it needs, and health problems declared "something you will just have to live with" will almost magically begin to disappear.

If you join the Weston A. Price Foundation, one wonderful thing they send you is their annual "Shopping Guide." This is a small pamphlet chock full of information on the best, most nutritionally dense foods to buy in different categories. That information alone is worth the cost of joining the foundation.

In trying to sort through all of the different views on nutrition – what is right, what is not – I decided to take a very unusual stand (for me at least) by looking at nature. What are different animals designed (or evolved) to eat, and what are we designed to eat? Cows eat grass – ideally pasture grass and not genetically modified corn products. Chickens in the wild eat more than grains; they eat a variety of organic material including insects and other high protein snacks. If you deny them these nutrients, their meat and products – such as their eggs and milk – will also be nutrient deficient.

The documentary *King Corn* states most beef in this country is fed corn meal from GMO corn. Several decades ago, it took a cow four to five years to reach a weight of 1,200 pounds, the weight when they are usually slaughtered. By switching from a natural grass diet to an exclusive corn-meal diet, this time can be reduced to only fourteen to sixteen months. But, it is at a cost, a cost to the health of the cow and a cost to the nutritional value and safety of the meat.

A cow's stomach is generally pH neutral. A diet of corn makes its stomach extremely acid and in doing so, the cow must be slaughtered before being on a corn diet 120 days. The cow also must be given antibiotics, protein supplements, and growth hormones. Eighty percent of the antibiotics produced in the United States go to the beef industry. Because of the high acid levels in their stomachs, corn-fed cows are prone to health issues such as bloat, diarrhea, ulcers, liver disease, and a weakened immune system. This leaves them in a state where E. coli can thrive. E. coli not only gets into the meat, it can also be transferred to the consumer and the results can then be fatal. [13]

It is best to buy produce and meats from local farmers and ranchers whenever possible. I live in Texas and there are many avenues to obtain these products. In more urban areas, it may require more effort, but start with your local Farmer's Market. Many ranchers now bring their meats, as well as fruits and vegetables, to the market. If you are unsure, consult the Weston A. Price website for more information in obtaining foods from the best sources possible.

Overall, organic foods contain fewer pesticides, they contain more omega-3 fats, and they contain less dangerous bacteria. Grass-fed beef contains four times the amount of vitamin E as corn-fed beef as well as significantly higher levels of calcium, magnesium, beta-carotene, and potassium. [14]

The ground in which industrial farmers grow vegetables is also stripped of proper nutrition. The organic materials needed to feed the soil have been ignored and now chemical fertilizers are sprayed on the earth. Vegetables are also often sprayed with herbicides to prevent the growth of weeds, which then disrupts the natural flora in our gut.

From everything I have read, I strongly believe a vegetarian and especially a vegan diet is not healthy. Our eye-teeth show we are designed by God or nature to eat meat. If we were supposed to solely eat vegetables, we would have a ruminant digestive system, like a cow. If you do have one of these, then by all means, become a vegan. If you don't, add quality, nutrient-dense meat to your diet. <u>Many nutrients our bodies require, such as vitamin B-12, thiamine, riboflavin, pantothenic acid, folate, niacin and vitamin B6, are available primarily through red meats.</u> I do, however, believe there may be short-term benefits to a purely vegan diet (one or two months), mainly because of certain detoxifying effects. A vegan diet is able to rapidly change a body's pH balance from acid to balanced or even slightly alkaline.

Probably my favorite story of nutritional density over adversity is the life of Dr. Terry Wahls. After receiving her medical degree, marriage and two children, she was diagnosed with an aggressive form of Multiple Sclerosis (MS). Within a short time, she could no longer walk and was confined to a reclining power chair. As a doctor, she tells, she had access to the best medicines, research, hospitals and other doctors, yet no one was able to help her. She took matters into her own hands and began eating a diet similar to mine, but with special focus on certain vegetable groups. She was able to completely reverse the symptoms of the disease. She is now free of her power chair and even bicycles competitively. Notice I didn't say she was "cured" of MS, only that she no longer has the debilitating symptoms. Her books are *Minding My Mitochondria* and *The Wahls Protocol* and I strongly recommend them for anyone suffering from MS, Parkinson's disease or Alzheimer's. [42]

Popular right now is the book, *The China Study* and the documentary *Forks Over Knives*. I do think a diet rich in vegetables is good for all of us, but what *The China Study* failed to mention is although deaths by heart disease may decline slightly, deaths by all other causes rise when eating a strictly vegetarian diet.

Another issue is fats, especially saturated fats. The US Government has done an excellent job over the last 50 years convincing us that animal fats are bad for us. Yet, as we have moved to a "fat-free" and vegetable oil existence, we have seen dramatic rises in heart disease, cancer, diabetes and obesity. As I said earlier, 100 years ago, only 1 person in 30 suffered from heart disease. Now that number is 1 in 3. We don't know the blood serum cholesterol numbers of people at that time, but what I do know with absolute certainty is that when they butchered a pig or cow, they did not select only the leanest cuts to eat. The entire animal was consumed. Nothing was wasted, including the organ meat. They drank only whole milk, never non-fat or low-fat. They ate butter from real cream, not butter substitutes made from GMO vegetable oils. Yet, they suffered far less problems with heart disease. They were also closer to their sources of food and processed, packaged food products had not yet been introduced.

There are a multitude of reasons our bodies need fat. This partial list is from the website *Empowered Sustenance*:

- Healthy Bile Release Requires Fat.
- Gallbladder Health Requires Fat.
- Fat-Soluble Vitamins are Found in Fat.
- Cholesterol Balance Requires Plenty of Good Fats.
- Blood Sugar Balance Requires Good Fats.
- Protein Utilization Requires Fat.
- Hormone Balance Requires Fat.
- Detox Requires Fat.
- Weight Loss and Weight Management Require fat.
- Fat Makes Food Taste Good.

The next step in this book is several steps combined, but all are on the same path. Seek the most nutrient dense foods possible, and your body with heal itself without other intervention.

STEP 18: BUY AND CONSUME NUTRIENT-DENSE FOODS

Drink Raw, Whole Milk from Grass-Fed Cows

Not only is raw, whole milk from grass-fed cows extremely nutrient dense, it also raises your body's pH acid level so that it is more alkaline. Hence, I could have also put this in *Part I* of this book.

I am defining raw milk as milk from cows that are fed only grass and the milk has not been pasteurized nor homogenized. Often these cows are allowed to graze freely in pastures.

I am always surprised at the shocked look on people's faces when I tell them I drink raw milk. The first questions always revolve around whether or not this is risky behavior. Nothing could be further from the truth. Whole, raw milk is nature's perfect, complete food. Once the milk is pasteurized and homogenized, many of the essential enzymes and nutrients are killed off. Even worse, the fat in milk is essential for your body to properly digest and process the rest of the milk.

When I was younger, I never heard of anyone being "lactose intolerant." Now it seems almost too common. Do you wonder why? As the government and dairies pushed low-fat and non-fat milks upon us as being "healthy," we lost the fat necessary to digest the milk. Milk then became an irritant to our stomach and bowels, and our bodies responded with an allergic reaction. By the way, drinking low-fat milk does not make you less fat any more than drinking diet soda makes you lose weight. Ingesting fat does not make you fat. Low-fat and non-fat milk are imbalanced foods. If you drink these, your body will react as if there is a food/fat shortage and begin saving other foods as fats. Sugars, chemical sugar substitutes and carbohydrates are what actually make you fat.

Interestingly, most people who have been labeled lactose intolerant, can drink raw, whole milk.

Milk is nature's perfect, complete food. Protests that adults should not be drinking milk are unfounded. I do agree that pasteurized, homogenized milk from confinement dairies of cows fed GMO corn meal is bad for us. But raw, whole milk from pasture or grass-fed cows is a nutritional powerhouse that shouldn't be ignored. One of my favorite protests against drinking milk is that "we are the only mammal which continues to drink milk past the infant stage" implying we shouldn't. I've got news for you all. We are the only mammals which clothe ourselves, the only mammals which cook our food, the only mammals which sow and reap. Should we not do those things either? This protest ignores the primary question: Is milk good for us? From multi-cultural health studies where the diet is primarily milk and milk products, the answer is a resounding yes.

Safety issues of raw milk are exaggerated as most pasteurized milk is produced in confinement dairies under filthy, inhumane conditions and cows regularly being injected with antibiotics, with the attitude "Hey, it's going to be pasteurized, so what difference does it make!" Most raw milk is produced from cows naturally grazing on pasture grasses. Grass-fed cows produce the healthiest milk and meat, especially pasture-fed (naturally grazing on grass out on a pasture). Avoid all cattle products from cows fed primarily corn.

The seminal book on this subject is *The Untold Story of Milk: The History, Politics and Science of Nature's Perfect Food* by Ron Schmid.

Because of laws in different states, raw milk is not easily available everywhere. In California, I was able to find it in two or three stores. Here in Texas, I had to join a co-op and I pick up my milk weekly. A great resource for information on obtaining raw milk in your area is the Weston A. Price Foundation website (www.westonaprice.org). For some reason, the Obama administration finds the sale of raw milk to be especially upsetting and has maintained a serious offensive against dairy farmers, often arresting them and dumping their inventory. Fortunately, Weston A. Price has a defense fund to help these farmers/ranchers, and in almost all cases, the charges are dropped or the farmers are found not guilty of any crime. I find it interesting that marijuana growers and smokers are celebrated these days while raw milk producers and drinkers are vilified!

Raw milk has also helped many couples overcome problems with conception. A neighbor of my aunt and uncle tried for years to get pregnant. The couple was about to go the expensive, fertility clinic route when my uncle suggested they both begin drinking raw milk daily. Within five months they were pregnant. This along with eliminating soy products should be the first thing any couple should try if they have problems with conception (See Step 6).

One question I am constantly asked is, "What does it taste like?" Well, it tastes like milk, very fresh milk. Once you drink it, you'll never drink the processed garbage again. If unable to obtain raw milk, try at least to get non-homogenized milk. The homogenization process also breaks down many of the essential nutrients and enzymes contained in milk. Be sure with raw milk or any non-homogenized milk to "shake before using."

When buying any dairy product, check the ingredients. Sour cream should be milk or cream and little else. Some brands are loaded with a variety of unnecessary and unhealthful additives. The same is also true of yogurt and cream cheese. Never buy any dairy product which has been "ultra-pasteurized." The product is subjected to such high heat that basically all nutritional value is eliminated. These milk products no longer even require refrigeration.

Also, the FDA has recently approved milk producers (confinement dairies producing pasteurized, homogenized milk) to add aspartame to sweeten milk without forcing them to prominently display "diet" or "lite" on the label. Since it is unlikely anyone would check milk for the sweeteners it contains, in my mind, this is the same as allowing aspartame to be added without having to label it. [41, 43]

We are artificially adding a chemical product in milk purportedly in the interest of "taste."

Eat Grass-Fed (Pasture-Fed) Beef

As I mentioned above, most beef is from cows fed a diet of GMO corn which is detrimental to the cow's health. Some markets and butchers are finally responding to consumer demand and are carrying grass-fed beef. Also, you can find ranchers in many areas who sell this type of beef, often at farmer's markets. It is more expensive, but you will be giving your body what it wants and needs. Go one step further and ask the farmer/store from which you are buying grass-fed beef for the bones, organ meats, and other parts of the cow that most people aren't looking to buy.

You can then use these parts to make homemade bone broth (See Step 21). You may even receive these items for free because most people don't ask for them. If not, you are likely to pay a very reasonable price for them.

Eat Organic, Free-Roaming Chicken

Note the size difference in chickens which are organic and free-roaming to standard, packaged chickens. I've seen packaged chicken breasts almost larger than entire organic chickens. It is amazing what can be accomplished through hormones and other unnatural processes. But this robs the meat and subsequently our bodies of essential nutrition.

Eat Eggs From Organic, Free-Roaming Chickens

When you buy eggs from organic, free-roaming chickens and break them open, the first thing you will notice is the deep yellow/orange color of the yolks. These are the eggs I remember as a child – deep in color and rich in nutrition – not the pale, unnatural color of most store-bought eggs. Not only are these eggs more nutritious, the chickens are raised under far more humane conditions. Try to find a local farm as a resource for eggs. Many eggs marked "free-roaming, organic" eked past the requirement by letting hundreds of chickens outside for an hour each day in small, fenced areas. As I mentioned before, if you join the Weston A. Price foundation you will receive a wonderful pocket shopping guide which will also list the brands of eggs which are especially nutritious.

If you are so inclined, the best option is to raise your own chickens in your yard. This is becoming more and more popular in the U.S., along with vegetable gardens. You then know exactly from where your food comes and the quality within.

Organic eggs provide a healthy source of cholesterol which is important for maintaining cell integrity. This helps to prevent cancer. Eggs contain the full spectrum of essential amino acids, the building blocks for protein. Eggs are also a good source of protein, fat, and carotenoids. The less your eggs are cooked, the more nutritious they are for you. I eat two raw organic eggs a day.

I addressed the arguments of "eggs have cholesterol" in my prior book. So, be sure to eat the entire egg, not merely the whites.

The yolks contain the bulk of the nutrition your body needs. If you are chasing cholesterol, you are not seeking health. Consume nutrient dense foods if you are seeking chronic good health.

The issue of cholesterol has also been addressed in many other excellent books including:

- *Statin Drugs Side-Effects and the Mis-Guided War on Cholesterol* by Dr. Duane Graveline.
- *The Great* Cholesterol *Myth* by Jonny Bowden and Steve Sinatra
- *Nourishing Traditions* by Sally Fallon
- *Malignant Medical Myths* by Joel M. Kauffman, Ph.D.

It is evident from reading these four books, that for women, it has been shown that the higher your cholesterol, the longer you will live. Statin drugs (cholesterol lowering drugs such as Lipitor or Crestor) are so dangerous they really should be banned. But, they are also over a $30 billion a year industry, so it will take a lot to get in front of that train. The FDA is now even considering putting statins into our water. Note also that there has never been a single study completed on statin drugs that used women as a test subject. Statin drugs have never been tested on women; yet, they are continuing to be prescribed on a daily basis. [26] It has also been shown that statins increase a woman's risk of breast cancer by over 200%. [34]

Eat Organic Vegetables

So much of our produce has been bastardized that it barely resembles food anymore. Most produce in our markets has been grown in soil which has been stripped of almost all nutrition. [15] Much of the produce has also been genetically modified and is loaded with herbicides.

The best source for organic vegetables is local farmer's markets. In your local market check the PLU codes on fruits and vegetables. Avoid any which start with the number "8" and try to buy only produce which starts with the number "9" which indicates it is organic.

The following are the produce you especially want to buy as organic as they tend to be especially dirty or contaminated:

- Apples
- Celery
- Cucumbers
- Grapes
- Bell peppers
- Cherry tomatoes
- Nectarines
- Kale
- Peaches
- Spinach
- Potatoes
- Strawberries

The better you eat, the better you will feel and the fewer ailments and disease you will have. Yes, it costs more, but so does medical treatment and time off work. For me, the trade-off seems obvious.

STEP 19: REPLACE ALL "BUTTER" SPREADS WITH REAL PASTURE BUTTER

The government and the food industries have worked relentlessly over the last 50 years to convince us that animal fats are bad for us. Nothing could be further from the truth. Our bodies require fats to function properly. The body requires real fats, not vegetable fats hydrogenated and processed into something attempting to be "real." Butter is packed with nutrition and fats needed by our bodies.

Butter contains lecithin and a number of anti-oxidants which protect against free radical damage that weakens the arteries. Vitamins A and E are also found abundantly in butter.

Butter also protects against arthritis, osteoporosis, varicose veins and heart disease.

I put butter on almost everything I eat.

Eating margarine can increase heart disease in women by 53% over eating the same amount of butter, according to a recent Harvard Medical Study. Margarine also triples the risk of coronary heart disease, increasing total cholesterol and LDL (the presently categorized "bad cholesterol") and lowering the HDL (the presently categorized "good cholesterol"). Margarine increases the risk of cancer by almost five times over butter.

Between 1920 and 1960, heart disease rose to become the number one killer in America. During that same time the consumption of butter went from 18 pounds per person per year to only 4. [16]

I love the line from the Swedish movie, *Pelle, The Conqueror* when Max von Sydow says to his grandson that in Denmark, life is so good that "they put butter on their bread an inch thick." I love the word "slather" when I put butter on foods. I think of the nutritional benefits of butter and always am saddened if I find I am served margarine or other butter substitutes in restaurants. At those places, I simply go without. At home, I have "pasture butter" on hand at all times. Pasture butter is labeled as such.

Margarine is so bad and so unlike food that, if left outside, even bugs won't eat it or even land on it. If bugs won't eat it, do you really want it in your body?

STEP 20: REPLACE GROCERY STORE "SALT" WITH ORGANIC, RAW SEA SALT

Much like fats, our bodies require salt to function. Sadly, the salt we find in our grocery stores has been processed to the point it no longer possesses any nutritional value. Seek out raw, unprocessed sea salt. I use Celtic salt harvested from the north of France by Eden Foods.

Sea Salt comes from natural sea water evaporated under the sun and contains five percent potassium and other minerals which give it its flavor. The minerals are readily absorbed and used by the body as they are naturally occurring.

Table salt is refined using high heat and chemicals. Potassium and sodium iodine are added into the salt and color is created using dextrose and sodium bicarbonate.

Another advantage of using real salt is that it is good for you and therefore, you shouldn't feel hesitant to use it. In using it, the real flavors of food will come out and you will feel satisfied. It will help you to stop using monosodium glutamate (MSG) or foods containing it. MSG has a similar effect on the body as aspartame (See *Step 2: Eliminate Sugar*).

MSG is hidden in many products and often under different names such as glutamic acid. Again, our friends in the FDA, in their continued attempts to protect us, do not require labeling of many products containing MSG. The list of processed foods clandestinely containing MSG is long and can be found on www.truthinlabeling.org .

Reduced salt intake does not lower blood pressure. Since the introduction of the myth that it does, many studies have been conducted in an attempt to prove this hypothesis. No study has shown this to be true other than lowering salt intake may *slightly* lower ones systolic pressure.

To get a more complete understanding of this issue, read Dr. David Brownstein's *Salt Your Way To Health.*

STEP 21: MAKE YOUR OWN BONE BROTH

Homemade bone broth is so good and so good for you. The broth you buy in the supermarket has almost no nutritional benefit and is loaded with non-natural salt. The reasons grandma's homemade chicken soup was so good and healing was because she started with a good chicken and she first made healthful bone broth. This broth is easy-to-make and delicious to taste.

The benefits include helping your body heal leaky gut, fight infections such as colds and flu, reduce joint pain and inflammation, improve skin, hair and nails; help with bone formation and repair, and promotion of good sleep. It is essential after any type of surgery or bone fracture to consume bone broth regularly.

I make both chicken and beef bone broth. My recipe is at the end of this book.

Bone broth is cooked slowly over a couple of days with the addition of raw, organic vinegar to pull the nutrients from the bones.

You do not need to use the broth only for soups; you can simply drink a small amount every day. If you do this, you will probably want to season it with organic, raw sea salt to bring out the flavor (something I do not add when making the broth).

This is another very easy step. I usually save the meat from the chicken and the beef and then make soup shortly after the broth is finished. The extra broth I freeze in 1 cup packets for other uses.

STEP 22: ELIMINATE ANYTHING MARKED "LOW FAT," "NON FAT," "LITE" OR "DIET"

Not only do our bodies need fat to function properly, the most disconcerting part of "low fat" or "diet" products is what is added to these items to qualify for that label. Good fats are removed and replaced with bad fats, such as vegetable oils, many having GMO origins.

"Diet" often means the addition of artificial chemical sweeteners like aspartame. These are often poisons your body doesn't need or want.

I love the quote from Joan Collins, "I don't drink diet soda because you never see skinny people drinking it!" Diet sodas and other diet processed foods do not make you skinny or keep you from getting fat or fatter, in fact, they seem to contribute to obesity.

We as a country will not become healthy until the myth that "fat is bad" is set aside. Fat is essential, but sugar and artificial chemical sweeteners truly are extremely bad for us.

To learn more about the dangers of artificial sweeteners, read this excellent article by Dr. Mercola [4].

PART IV

Vitamins and Supplements

> *"One of the first duties of the physician is to educate the masses not to take medicine."*
>
> -Dr. William Osler

For years, doctors have told us that we get all the nutrition we need from our diet. That may have been true 150 years ago, but it is definitely NOT true today. Our food has been stripped of nutrition, most frequently, in the interest of longer shelf life or because of processing the foods.

I am limiting the number of vitamins and other nutrients (e.g. minerals) I am recommending, focusing primarily on those most Americans, or those eating an American diet, are especially deficient. These deficiencies often lead to chronic diseases.

As I listen to commercials for various prescription drugs and their long lists of warnings, often including death, I can't help wonder why people are so resistant to taking vitamins, minerals and organic foods yet so ready and willing to take another drug.

In general, buy nutrients in capsule form. Tablets often contain binders and fillers and are compressed under tremendous pressure, often making them difficult to break down in our digestive systems. It is usually best to take vitamins with food (especially fat soluble vitamins) unless otherwise instructed.

You will probably want to keep your doctor(s) informed of the nutrients you are taking. If he tells you to stop taking them, ask for the "peer-reviewed, double-blind studies" that states taking the specific nutrients are bad for you. If he gets angry or refuses, take that as a sign he really knows nothing about your specific health path.

I know many people are confused as to which brands of vitamins are best and which are worst. In general, never buy from chain drug stores or large box stores. I have been a member of the Life Extension Foundation for over twenty years. I know I may not be getting the *highest* quality, but I am getting a very good quality product. (www.lef.org). If you join the Life Extension Foundation you will receive a very informative monthly magazine with the latest research in alternative health therapy. I often repost articles from their website onto my blog.

I do recommend taking a good multi-vitamin as well. Do not buy your multi-vitamins from large chain drug stores or large box stores. Never buy any brand which has its own television commercial. They provide doses of the vitamins so low they will do your body little or no good.

I suggest the following. If nothing else, compare what you look for against the nutrient levels in this supplement: Two-Per-Day Capsules from *Life Extension.* [17]

STEP 23: TAKE MAGNESIUM OIL

Most Americans are deficient in magnesium. Our sugar- and carbohydrate-rich diets deplete our bodies of this essential mineral. Low magnesium leads to improperly absorbed calcium (which then leads to osteoporosis), difficulty sleeping, high blood sugar levels, headaches, migraines and the list goes on and on. Magnesium helps to prevent heart attacks, high blood pressure, and heart arrhythmia.

If there is only one thing you take from this book, start using magnesium oil (usually the oils contain magnesium chloride, probably the most effective form of magnesium). Considering the immune enhancing properties of magnesium, it is important for optimal health, regardless of your own health objectives in reading this book.

Magnesium is a cellular detoxifier and tissue purifier and is necessary for many enzyme reactions. Most cancer patients have very low levels of cellular magnesium, so adding magnesium to your regimen also works as a cancer inhibitor. It greatly improves immune functions and reduces pain. Cells not getting enough magnesium will die. Proper levels of magnesium are essential for strong bones and teeth, balanced hormones and a healthy nervous and cardiovascular system. Magnesium helps turn food into energy and keeps muscles from cramping. It also decreases insulin resistance.

Magnesium plays a role in over 300 enzyme reactions in the body and is necessary for protein formation and DNA production.

I recommend Ancient Minerals' magnesium oil available on the internet (the link is provided at the end of this book). You spritz 10 to 15 shots of it on your skin, rubbing it in with your inner arm. If you find it causes a mild burning sensation, you can wash it off after 20 minutes.

It takes about three to four months of using this product to increase your cellular levels of magnesium, but it is worth the wait and the cost.

It takes 287 molecules of magnesium to metabolize just one single molecule of glucose. So, do <u>you</u> think you are you getting enough magnesium?

For more information on magnesium and its health benefits, visit the Weston A. Price website (<u>www.westonaprice.org</u>) or read *The Magnesium Miracle* by Caroline Dean, M.D. N.D.

STEP 24: TAKE IODINE

Iodine is one of the most important things you can add to your nutritional regimen, especially if you live in the Great Lakes region of the United States. For some reason, iodine levels are especially low in the surrounding areas, and the population there is especially deficient.

Iodine is necessary for life. It is contained in each cell of our bodies. Iodized salt from the supermarket is a joke. It supplies neither the proper type of iodine nor sufficient daily levels. Through food, the average Japanese adult consumes approximately 13 milligrams (or 13,000 micrograms) of iodine per day from their diet. Doctors in the U.S. say anything over 500 micrograms daily is "dangerous" and can lead to iodine "poisoning."

To relieve you of any fears that higher doses will "poison" you, know that I and at least five people I know take over 50 milligrams of iodine per day with no adverse effects.

The best form in which to take iodine is Lugol's Solution (a blend of Potassium Iodide and Iodine). You can easily find this on the Internet, including Amazon.com, from various companies.

You can either add drops of the solution to water and drink or apply it to your skin and let your body absorb it. Iodine does stain but disappears over time. Do not use the palms of your hands to rub in the iodine since you are apt to wash your palms throughout the day. Use instead, the inside of your lower arm. I usually apply it to my thigh or stomach.

The consummate guide on iodine is Dr. David Brownstein's book, *Iodine: Why You Need It and Why You Can't Live Without It.*

Iodine helps prevent many forms of cancer, especially thyroid, breast, ovarian, prostate and testicular cancers. According to Dr. Brownstein, he has also had tremendous success reversing fibrocystic disease in women's breasts.

Iodine often reverses a host of seemingly unrelated illnesses in the upper torso, any area near the thyroid. My cousin found that iodine reversed her frozen shoulder problem.

This step (Iodine) along with Magnesium Oil, are the two steps you should implement as quickly as possible.

STEP 25: TAKE COD LIVER OIL

Cod liver oil provides vitamins A and D, both which are fat soluble. Dr. Weston A. Price found that primitives, people belonging to preliterate, nonindustrial society or culture, consumed levels of A and D ten times higher than in our modern diet and they were far healthier than we are today. Many of the chronic conditions we experience were non-existent at that time. Cod liver oil also contains high levels of DHA and EPA, both essential for proper functioning of the brain and nervous system. Diabetics can especially benefit from taking daily doses of cod liver oil.

Cod liver oil should be purchased in dark bottles and stored in dark, cool places. Ideally, it should be fermented. Just as your grandmother thought, cod liver oil, in small doses, is an excellent supplement for growing children.

What about cod liver oil versus other fish oils? I have read some articles from trusted sources saying krill oil is even better. But I know many fish oils are extruded under high heat which may destroy and negate many of their benefits.

"Fermented cod liver oil" is processed under low heat and the fermentation preserves the nutritional value of the product. I especially recommend Green Pastures Blue Ice Royal Butter Oil/Fermented Cod Liver Oil Blend.

Cod liver oil should be taken by women suffering from pre-menstrual syndrome (PMS). It can ease symptoms such as cramping, tenderness, bloating and headaches. It is also important for women who suffer from PMS to take magnesium and additional calcium (preferable calcium citrate).

Cod liver oil is also excellent at helping prevent tooth decay. Read *Cure Tooth Decay: Heal and Prevent Cavities with Nutrition* by Ramiel Nagel for more information on the amazing properties of this oil and what other steps you can do to treat tooth problems naturally.

If you simply cannot handle the taste, try Carlson's Soft Gel 1,000 milligram Capsules (as I do).

STEP 26: TAKE VITAMINS D3, K2, NIACIN AND VITAMIN B-12

I have selected these four vitamins because they seem to be especially deficient from the American diet and the ailments associated with these deficiencies are becoming more and more common.

Vitamin D3

It has been decided by the powers that be that the sun is our enemy; we shouldn't go out into the sun for even a moment without first slathering ourselves with sun screen. Yet our bodies need sunlight. With the sun, our bodies are able to manufacture Vitamin D which is essential for proper calcium absorption and also for a sense of well-being. Many people who suffer from depression have found by simply supplementing their diets with Vitamin D3, the fog begins to lift. Ideally, spending time in the sun is best, but in many climates, this is simply not possible during the winter months.

D3 is also essential for our bodies to process and absorb calcium. Is it any wonder we have seen a rise in bone fractures in the elderly during the same time we've told people to avoid the sun? I agree that spending hours and hours, day after day in the sun is probably not good for anyone, but hiding inside and overusing sun screen takes its toll as well.

If you cannot get out into the sun, supplement your diet with at least 1,000 to 5,000 IUs (international units) per day of vitamin D3.

Vitamin K2

Along with Vitamin D3, K2 is vital for proper calcium absorption from the foods we eat. Without it, the body will scavenge itself, usually from our bones and teeth, for the calcium it needs to function properly. K2 deficiency leads to osteoporosis, varicose veins, arterial calcification, cardiovascular disease, as well as prostate, lung and liver cancers. Along with Vitamin D3, low levels of K2 can also lead to Parkinson's disease. Take at least

1,000 mcgs of Vitamin K2 per day. If you suffer from Parkinson's disease, I would probably double that amount.

There are also multiple anti-cancer properties of K2, especially regarding liver cancer. [18]

Niacin (Vitamin B3)

Niacin deficiency can lead to many of the same problems as Vitamin D deficiency – especially when it comes to mental health. One recent documentary I watched talked of an elderly woman living with her children and grandchildren. She became so depressed she did nothing but sit in the dining room, facing the wall all day long. She did not interact with anyone in the family.

A naturopath told the family to give her niacin and as much as was necessary. They began giving it to her, slowly increasing the dose. Around 5,000 mgs, the woman responded and rejoined the family. She was her "old self" again. That is, until she visited her family doctor and, when she told him of her "solution," he replied "Wow, that is a really big dose of niacin. I'm not sure that is a good idea!" It scared the woman, so she stopped. Within days, she was back in the corner, staring at the wall.

We also know of niacin's helpful effects on reducing cholesterol levels. I do not believe in chasing cholesterol numbers, so this is of no interest to me. (For more information on this, read, *Statin Drugs, Side Effects and the Misguided War on Cholesterol* by Dr. Duane Graveline.) But, if you disagree and want to reduce your cholesterol numbers, try starting with a dose of about 500 mgs of niacin daily (taken with a meal). You will likely feel a flushing sensation after taking it, but it will pass. Slowly increase the dose, over several weeks, to 2,500 to 3,000 mgs. Doses of niacin higher than 2,200 mgs increases HDL, increases the particle size of LDL and reduces triglycerides.

In the Coronary Drug Project study, niacin was shown to reduce the risk of non-fatal heart attacks and strokes by 27% and 26% respectively. Study participants were all survivors of prior heart attacks. [19]

Vitamin B-12

Vitamin B-12 is an essential nutrient and one in which vegetarians are often deficient. It is not easily absorbed through the stomach, so it is best to take this either by injection or sublingually (a tablet dissolved under the tongue). Improving gut health through the steps in Part II of this book will also help with vitamin B-12 absorption through the foods you eat, especially red meat. The best form to take vitamin B-12 is as methylcobalamin.

A good friend was recently asked by her doctor if she was diabetic. Although she exhibits many of the symptoms, she told him she had been tested repeatedly and was not. But, she had numbness in her toes or peripheral neuropathy, a symptom often associated with diabetes. If the situation becomes too dire and blood flow is cut off, it can result in amputation. But this doctor, thankfully, looked further and tested her vitamin B-12 levels. They were found to be unusually low and the numbness went away after a B-12 shot.

If you find yourself always tired and lacking energy, this would be the first thing I would suggest trying.

For more information read *Vitamin B-12 for Health* by Dr. David Brownstein

STEP 27: TAKE COQ10

With the massive push in the pharmaceutical industry to expand the use of cholesterol-lowering statin drugs, the natural process in our bodies that statins interrupt also stops the production of the essential nutrient Coenzyme Q10.

Deficiencies in CoQ10 lead to heart disease, heart failure, and cancer. In one Japanese study, patients who took doses of CoQ10 of over 200 mgs per day dramatically reduced their risks of heart attack. My own blog has an article on using CoQ10 for cancer treatment. [20]

In ranking of steps to take in this book, I would rank this one in the top five. But, be sure you take at least 200 to 400 mgs per day; lower doses have minimal effect on the body. Also be sure to take CoQ10 in the ubiquinol form instead of the more common ubiquinone.

High doses of CoQ10 have also been shown to slow the progression of Parkinson's Disease in studies conducted by the Life Extension Foundation. Because CoQ10 is an essential component of healthy mitochondrial function, it also helps with reducing effects of Multiple Sclerosis.

PART V:

Toxins

As you look through this list of toxins, note I don't list "Eliminate Smoking" as a step. I hope those of you reading this book already know that smoking is extremely unhealthful. On the other hand, a study by Dr. Broda Barnes also showed that a properly functioning body can even negate most of the negative effects of something as dangerous and unhealthful as smoking.

Toxins are everywhere in our lives. Ideally, move away from urban areas where the concentration of smog is highest, grow your own vegetables, raise your own chickens and cows, and plant fruit trees. This is more than most people can do, so I have listed some of the most common and dangerous toxins to which most Americans expose themselves daily.

Toxins pop up in some of the most surprising places. I was reading an article recently that many brands of balsamic vinegar contain lead. I was stunned. I like the taste of that vinegar and use it often. I went to check my bottle on the shelf and sure enough, "Contains Lead" was on the label. I couldn't help but wonder how something as toxic as lead could be in any food product sold in the U.S. I immediately poured the vinegar down the drain and found another brand without the warning. Now, I have also read that all balsamic vinegars contain trace amounts of lead. So, even what I bought may be tainted. This means I will use it sparingly.

There are many other toxins to which we are exposed daily. I cannot begin to list them all, but these are some of the most common and easily eliminated from our homes and our lives.

STEP 28: ELIMINATE SODIUM FLUORIDE

Sodium Fluoride is an industrial waste product that is also used as rat poison. It supposedly prevents cavities, although no study has ever shown this to be true, other than in places where their water naturally contains fluoride (not Sodium Fluoride). Check the label on your toothpaste tube and note the warning about ingesting it. It is a poison and has no place anywhere in your body. [36]

Most non-English speaking countries reject water fluoridation and recently Israel has reversed their decision to fluoridate water. This is based on a lack of evidence it does any good and evidence it is actually harmful.

I use a brand of toothpaste called "Desert Essence," although there are now (thankfully) several brands of fluoride-free toothpaste from which to choose. You can also make your own toothpaste from coconut oil, baking soda, diatomaceous earth, and other natural ingredients. Check the internet for various recipes, if interested. A simple tooth powder recipe is included at the back of this book.

STEP 29: ELIMINATE MERCURY

Do a search on the internet regarding mercury poisoning and the effects on the human body. Yet somehow, someway, according to our government, this highly toxic poison is perfectly acceptable in an amalgam in our teeth! Thankfully, many dentists have seen the light and no longer use amalgam in their practices, but many still tell us it is perfectly safe.

In the excellent documentary *A Beautiful Truth*, they show a tooth which was implanted with a mercury amalgam filling over 50 years prior. The mercury vapor is still clearly visible rising from the tooth and at a concentration that would cause a building to be evacuated. Yet here they are in our mouths.

Mercury poisoning first causes sensory impairment in vision, hearing and speech and also lack of coordination and tremors. Long exposure can cause death. [37]

Interestingly, just before the publication of this book I had a long chat with my dentist about mercury amalgam fillings. He said the official line is that no study has shown a link between the fillings and any illness. But, there is no question the mercury continually leaches out of the fillings and into our bodies. I'd like to ask any person conducting those studies if they would be willing to weekly drink a glass of water contaminated with mercury, assuring them, of course, that some researcher deemed it perfectly safe. Mercury is a poison and should not be in our bodies.

If you have mercury amalgam fillings, get them removed immediately and preferably by a dentist who is specially trained in this. One indicator is whether or not he has you prepare for the removal before ever coming into the office. Ideally they will suggest taking high doses of Vitamin C as well as Chlorella before and after the office visit. If they say any of this is nonsense, quickly find another dentist.

Mercury is one of the principle causes of heart failure. For some reason, mercury tends to settle in our heart muscle. If you have had amalgam fillings for quite some time and especially if you have any early stages of heart failure, you need to get on a regimen of chlorella tablets and high doses of Vitamin C. The mercury will bond to the chlorella and will help get some of the poison out of your system.

Of course, another dangerous source of mercury is vaccines where it is used as a preservative. It is banned in many countries, but not in all states in the United States. I take no vaccines and I find it alarming the magnitude of the increase in the number of vaccines the U.S. Government suggests we take over the last twenty-five years. From an adult standpoint, a few years ago it was merely the annual flu shot (which numbers even from the CDC show having minimal effect) but now it is for whooping cough, hepatitis, pneumonia, shingles and it seems as if the list continues to grow. There is a lot of profit in vaccines and minimal testing is done regarding their safety and efficacy. So how much mercury is in a typical flu shot vaccine? Using parts per billion (PPB) to measure levels, water is considered safe if it has less than 2 PPB, waste is considered hazardous if it has over 200 PPB, the typical flu shot has 50,000 PPB of mercury. These numbers are staggering yet the US Government, Big Pharmaceuticals and the AMA insist the vaccines are perfectly safe. If you take multiple vaccines in one year, think of the risk to which you subject yourself. [28, 29]

Do you know what happens to unused flu vaccine in Wisconsin? It needs to be treated at a hazardous waste collection site due to the huge amount of mercury it contains. In fact, it is 250 times higher than what is classified as hazardous waste. [28]

The following is from the Weston A. Price website:

Not only has there never been a single long-term study comparing the health and welfare of vaccinated to unvaccinated children, multiple examples can easily be found of vaccinated children acquiring the very illness they have been vaccinated against. Furthermore, there is overwhelming evidence that vaccines can be extremely harmful, permanently disabling and even deadly to our children. And the current system for tracking and reporting adverse reactions to the FDA is sloppy, poorly executed and voluntary rather than mandatory, even when a child has been permanently disabled or killed by a vaccine. [21]

If you feel the need to take vaccines, do not take multiple vaccines. If necessary, spread them out over time.

England recently settled a law suit against Glaxo Smith Kline over their swine flu vaccine which caused permanent brain damage in many of those who took it, both adults and children. [22]

With this in mind, remember it is recommended children receive 31 vaccinations before the age of four. That's a lot of mercury pumped into such a young system.

Also, avoid canned tuna as it is almost all contaminated with mercury. [23]

STEP 30: ELIMINATE ALUMINUM

As common as aluminum is in our modern homes, it too is neurotoxic and shows up in many unexpected places. There is evidence the long-term exposure is a factor in many diseases such as dementia, autism, and Parkinson's disease. [38]

Almost all antiperspirants contain aluminum. I want all women to think about this: just next to your breasts, you are applying a known poison daily, which is absorbed by your skin. I'm not saying aluminum containing antiperspirants cause cancer, but I am not saying it is safe for you either.

I have found a wonderful, natural, safe product from a small company in Florida called Primal Pit Paste. You can go to their website and order their products (they are also referenced in the back of this book). They are so safe, they are even edible.

Also check your baking powder. Many brands contain aluminum, although some, thankfully, do not.

Many brands of cheap cookware are made from aluminum, so every time you cook, the poisonous metal is getting into the food you eat. Some high-end brands claim they are perfectly safe, but then, many dentists claim mercury fillings are perfectly safe too.

I would rather be really safe than really sorry. I used to have the high-end aluminum cookware and got rid of it all when I had heart failure, spending hundreds of dollars on new stainless steel cookware. Also avoid cookware that is non-stick. [24]

PART VI
Other Voices

I have asked others who I admire to write a section in this book on topics I did not already cover. Each is important in its own way. Depending on whether you are maintaining good health or seeking answers to a chronic problem will probably determine how you use or view these steps.

Thank you to my contributors – each is special to me and each has a perspective I admire.

STEP A: MOVE EVERY SINGLE DAY

by Ashley Wise, MS CPT PNC

Move every single day. I am sure that this is not a new concept to you, and you might even be annoyed at hearing it yet again, but I want to encourage you to look at it from a different perspective.

The average person wakes up, gets ready for work, sits in their car or on a bus for the daily commute to work, walks to their desk where they sit for extended hours at time with a possible walking break to and from the rest room or the break room to refill their coffee or grab something to eat, back to their commute where they sit on their way home to sit down and eat dinner, and lastly top off their night with sitting on the couch to watch TV or in the stands to watch their child play sports or perform music. On a good day, this average person will get in 3,000+ steps - making it just above the half-way point of what classifies someone as 'sedentary'.

Now perhaps this isn't you. You are one of the few who make the commitment to go to the gym 3-5 times per week, or maybe even every single day. You carve out the hour or so to hit up the treadmill, elliptical or weights, feeling good that you have gotten in your daily exercise. You, my friend, dedicated to your daily workout, have done something great for your body and are more than likely sitting around 7,000 steps for your total day. Certainly not a bad place to be standing, yet you are still placed in the 'low active' category.

Low active?! But I go to the gym for an hour every day! How can I be told I am in the 'low active' category?

Let's look at this from a math perspective. There are 7 days in a week and 24 hours in a day, giving us 168 hours in a week. Exercising an hour in a given day, gives a person who works outs 3-7 days, 3-7 hours of activity in a given week. Or in other words, 0.2% - 0.4% of their week is spent being active.

But how can I add in more scheduled activity time? I have to work, sleep, spend time with my family, etc. I just don't see how I can add more exercise in!

And that is precisely why this step is titled Move Every Single Day, instead of "Exercise More Every Single Day."

The time you dedicate to exercising, whether it be running, strength training, doing yoga or crossfit, whatever it may be, is great. In fact, I highly encourage you to continue doing that and to continue to strive for improvements, it is one of the best things that you can be doing for your body and for your health. But it does not, and cannot, replace to being active overall.

A graduated step index for healthy adults released in 2004 states that less than 5000 steps per day classifies someone as "sedentary;" 5,000-7,499 steps per day as 'low active'; 7,500-9,999 steps per day as "somewhat active;" 10,000-12,500 steps per day as "active;" and more than 12,500 steps per day as "highly active."

In other words, to be considered 'active overall', an adult needs to be reaching a minimum of 10,000 steps per day.

Now this isn't 10,000 steps so that you can lose weight or tone up, although that could be a side effect depending on how many steps you are averaging in a day right now, but this is 10,000 steps to better your health and prevent onset of disease and illness.

People who average 10,000 steps per day decrease their chance of developing cardiovascular disease, coronary heart disease, type II diabetes, increased body mass index (BMI), depression, poor quality of life, high blood pressure, low HDL levels, an elevated waist circumference, high triglycerides, and elevated glucose values...and those are only a few of the added benefits!

To optimize the activity you are doing each day I do suggest investing in a pedometer. It doesn't need to be anything fancy, it just needs to count your steps. However, I do suggest the Fitbit. I am not affiliated with their company, I simply love their product. They have a variety of models to choose from, a great online data base, and will automatically upload your information to an iPhone or Android with their free app.

I know that it may seem impossible to reach 10,000 steps in a given day, but by focusing on altering or adding in a few minor things in your day, you will be amazed at how quickly the steps can add up.

Ways you can increase your daily steps:

- Park further away from the entrance
- Take the stairs
- Use a bathroom that is further away from your desk
- If possible, have walking meetings instead of boardroom meetings
- Vacuum your home more often than usual
- Schedule 10- to 15-minute breaks in your calendar throughout your day to get up and walk around
- Use your lunch break to go on a walk
- Start an after dinner walk tradition with your family
- Walk around at your child's events instead of sitting and watching
- Use the time in-between drop-off and pick-up for your children's event to get in a walk instead of running another errand
- Have walking coffee dates instead of coffee shop, coffee dates.

STEP B: SUNSHINE BENEFITS – DON'T BE AFRAID OF THE SUN!

by Kelly Moeggenborg aka Kelly the Kitchen Kop

It's spring and time to get out into the sunshine, right? Not according to some who say we should strictly limit our time in the sun, or that we should slather on plenty of sunscreen first to avoid wrinkles and skin cancer. But *how natural is that*? Sunscreen, full of nasty chemicals vs. sunshine, which helps our bodies make plenty of vitamin D...

Don't be afraid of the sun!

A COMMON SENSE ARTICLE FROM HARVARD MEDICAL SCHOOL

In recent years, the advice to totally avoid sun exposure hasn't set right with me. Yes, I know that some say there have been changes in the earth's ozone, so the sun can be more dangerous than in years past. But how could something as natural as the sun be unhealthy as many would have us believe? This article from Harvard Medical School on sunshine takes a more believable middle road on the issue:

- *"Several studies have suggested that suddenly getting a lot of sun is more dangerous than steady exposure over time."*
- *"There is a well-documented relationship between low vitamin D levels and poor bone health. Now links have been made to everything from multiple sclerosis to prostate cancer. "Linking" low vitamin D with these diseases doesn't prove cause-and-effect, but it suggests that possibility. Getting some sun may also shake off the wintertime blues: Research suggests that light hitting your skin, not just your eyes, helps reverse seasonal affective disorder (SAD). Moreover, being outside gets us golfing, gardening, and engaging in other types of physical activity."*

91

- *"Nobody wants to get skin cancer, but we've gone from sun worship to sun dread. Dr. Stern and others say there is a middle way that includes using a sunscreen with a sun protection factor (SPF) of at least 15 when you're outside for an extended period and wearing a hat and shirt around midday. So when summer's here, get outside and enjoy it!"*

MORE ON VITAMIN D AND THE MANY HEALTH BENEFITS:

- Prevents/treats depression and the "winter blues"/S.A.D. (Seasonal Affective Disorder)
- U.S. News and World Report: "Almost everyone needs more of the sunshine vitamin" – Vitamin D for bone health, lower diabetes risk, protection against TB, colds and flu
- Decreases multiple sclerosis risk
- Prevents cancer:

  1. Fox News: "Scientists Say Sunshine May Prevent Cancer"
  2. "Vitamin D Benefits from Sun Exposure Outshine Cancer Risk"
  3. USA Today: "Vitamin D research may have doctors prescribing sunshine" *The research of Dr. Edward Giovannucci, a Harvard University professor of medicine and nutrition, suggests that vitamin D might help prevent 30 deaths for each one caused by skin cancer. "I would challenge anyone to find an area or nutrient or any factor that has such consistent anti-cancer benefits as vitamin D," Giovannucci told the cancer scientists. "The data are really quite remarkable."*

HERE'S WHAT OUR FAMILY DOES:

As soon as there's a hint of spring in the air, we're outside as much as possible and our skin slowly builds up a good base. As we go through the summer, we rarely need much sunscreen. I only put it on the kids or I if we're going to be outside without shelter for a long time, especially in the middle of the day, or if we'll be by water, and then only after we get some sun without sunscreen for a while first. (How long depends on how much we've already been in the sun that year.) Sometimes I'll only put it on their cheeks, noses, shoulders and tops of their ears. You have to know your/your kid's skin and just be smart about it.

BE CAREFUL WITH THIS!

Use common sense. Be especially careful with kids. If your skin is very fair you may have to use more sunscreen than our family does. (Or if you haven't been in the sun much, and obviously if you're vacationing in a hotter climate.) Remember, the goal is to get some sunshine on your skin for the vitamin D (and probably many other health benefits that only God knows), but NEVER LET YOURSELF BURN!

WHAT ABOUT WRINKLES?

Most people think wrinkles are from sun damage. This may be partially true, and mostly if your skin has been burned a lot, but there are many other risk factors: age, smoking, stress, genetics, and I've also read that not getting enough <u>healthy fats</u> in your diet plays a HUGE role.

ALL NATURAL SUNSCREENS?

There are many non-toxic sunscreens on the market that have natural ingredients, so you can avoid the chemicals. We just use the cheap ones, though, because we really don't use it enough to justify the extra expense – they're very pricey. However, if you have very fair skin and/or you are in the sun a lot, it may be worth it to you.

WHO TO BELIEVE?

There are conflicting studies (big surprise!), and some sources still say that *any* sun exposure is dangerous. Do some reading and decide for yourself, but as always, above all, use common sense.

- The best way to get vitamin D in the winter: cod liver oil! (Don't worry, you can take the capsules.)
- Dr. Eades says the same thing, I love him!
- Omega 3's in cod liver oil can prevent sunburn – scroll down about 2/3 on this page to read about that and more on the many benefits of cod liver oil.
- Where is the TRUTH on health & nutrition?
- Last week's Rookie Tip: do you eat enough eggs?
- Need some meatless/vegetarian meal ideas?
- Other main dish ideas (scroll down through them all)

STEP C: CHIROPRACTIC AND YOUR HEALTH

by Dr. Kevin Farrar, D.C.

Why should Chiropractic be a part of your life? When it comes to Chiropractic many people are in the dark about what Chiropractic is, or what a Chiropractor does. When people think Chiropractic, the first thing they typically think is neck pain, back pain and headaches, they think twisting, popping and cracking bones and joints. I am going to explain what Chiropractic is and how much deeper it really goes. Chiropractors help people heal naturally without the use of drugs or surgery. This section is going to teach you what Chiropractic is and what you have been missing if Chiropractic is not already a part of your life.

To understand Chiropractic and how it can help you and your family you first have to understand what a Chiropractor does and why. Chiropractors specialize in the spine and nervous system because we understand if the brain and body are not properly communicating then it is impossible for your body to operate correctly. Chiropractors are experts in identifying nerve compression, irritation and injury within the spine. These problems can lead to devastating effects throughout the body as vital nerve signals are blocked or altered. These nerve impingements often start out very small and build over time, often being present for years or decades before symptoms show up.

Where do these nerve impingements come from and why they are there, may be your next thought. Throughout our life time we will encounter thousands of opportunities for our spine to become misaligned and damaged. When we are born our small developing spine goes through a large amount of trauma during the birth process, then in the process of learning to walk we fall between two to four thousand times. That doesn't stop us, we then start to play sports, ride bikes and climb trees, and of course we crash our bikes, we sometimes fall from where we are climbing and often encounter impacts while playing sports. When you think back on your youth it's sometimes a wonder how we survived to adult hood. When you stop and realize all your body has been through it's easy to see how we could have shifted our spine out of alignment in one or multiple places in just our youth alone.

In our adult years we will still have slips and falls, but we also have some new stresses that aren't typical in our youth. The biggest one being auto mobile accidents. The average person gets in an auto accident once every ten years. These impacts can be quite trivial or very life changing, but it is important to understand that any car accident over ten miles per hour is enough to cause a shift or even damage in our spine. Repetitive postures are often a huge problem for our adult population this is due to required use of computers in our work place. Ergonomics has become a big business and with great reason. We now understand the devastating effects of poor computer posture after five, ten, even twenty or more years. We have learned as we put the same stress on our body day in and day out without any effort to rebalance our body we will suffer in time.

Now you should be starting to understand how our body can become misaligned but what does that mean, where does pain come in to play, and how does all of this affect your health? Our spine is designed to protect our spinal cord and spinal nerves, but at the same time our spine also has to allow us to move, bend and twist. This is where the problems are created; as our spine is shifted out of position it starts to pinch the nerves that exit at that level of the spine. We have twenty four bones in our spine and we have nerves that exit on each side of each of those bones. These nerves carry our brain's vital messages out to our organs, our muscles and every cell in the body. At the same time those nerves are carrying information back from the body to the brain. The problems caused by spinal misalignments very greatly depending on what level in the spine is being compressed, what part of the nerve is being compressed, how severe the compression is as well as how long the problem has been present. These problems are also complicated by the health of the joints, bones and discs in this area.

Pain is a small part of the signals your nerves carry; only ten percent of your spinal nerves carry pain, the other ninety percent carries information for your muscles and organs. This can help you understand how nerve pressure can build up before you have any pain at all. Often time's pain is the very last signal to show up after your nerve pressure has developed to a point to where pain is caused. By this time other symptoms are likely present that you would have never related to nerve pressure within your spine.

The reason Chiropractors are thought of as neck, back or headache pain doctors is because Chiropractors are great at helping people reduce their pain, improve their function and their health. When you start to understand how the body works it makes great sense how Chiropractic helps the body. The symptoms we experience in our body are not accidental, or for no reason they ultimately have to be caused by some problem within the body. Chiropractors work to determine the root cause of each person's health problem and address what is causing the symptoms. When the problem is corrected the symptoms will leave because they are no longer being caused.

When it comes to Chiropractic the problems are spinal misalignments and nerve compression. The term for this is spinal subluxation. Once a person's subluxations are identified through examination and x-rays Chiropractors use gentle adjustments to guide the bone back into its correct position to allow the body to heal. The health of the joint as well as the length of time that person was subluxated will determine how long it takes for this area to return to health and stay there. Your Chiropractor will help you find a course of action necessary to retrain your spine to hold its proper alignment alleviating the problems caused by the nerves that were pinched by that bone.

Common symptoms people come to a Chiropractors office with are: neck pain, back pain, headaches, numbness in the arms or legs, weakness in the arms or legs, tension in the neck, back or shoulders, this is because these are common symptoms that develop from spinal subluxations. There is also a large portion of Chiropractic patients who come to a Chiropractor because they are having other dysfunction within their body such as digestive problems, hormone problems, neurological problems, thyroid problems, etc. Chiropractic can help these people as well if they have nerve compression that is affecting the area of their symptoms. Chiropractic is not the solution to every single problem and it is important to understand this is the reason for your exam and x-rays, this helps your Chiropractor determine if your complaint can be helped with Chiropractic or if you need a referral to another type of doctor.

The most important part of Chiropractic care as with any other type of health care is prevention. The best time to go to your dentist is not when your teeth fall out, nor is it the best time to see your optometrist when you are blind. You go to these doctors to prevent issues with your teeth and eyes and to maintain their health. Chiropractic is the same way; the best time to see a Chiropractor is when you are healthy or when you are not experiencing symptoms this will allow you to stay that way. Chiropractors do recommend maintenance visits in order to help you keep your spine and spinal nerves healthy. Just like your dentist recommends cleanings and checkups to prevent tooth decay and gum disease.

Prevention is essential because spinal health is a major problem in our society. Spinal disorders are the number one reason for functional disability in adults over the age of fifty. A functional disability is a problem that prevents a person from being able to move, work, and live as they normally would. When our joints are out of alignment, they wear unevenly. A common misconception is that arthritis and poor joint health are just part of getting older. This is only true if you do nothing to maintain your joint's health throughout your life time. Just like gum disease and tooth decay are only normal for people who do not brush their teeth, and go to their dentist.

If you want to experience a life of optimal health, not only living free of pain but being healthy then Chiropractic is an essential part of living that way. Chiropractors' help the body heal naturally and function at its best because we focus on helping patients find the root causes of their problems.

PART VII
Balancing Hormones

This is the only section which may require a visit to your doctor. Unless your hormones are in balance, almost nothing else you do will make you feel and be well. The endocrine system is vital to proper function of our bodies and especially our immune system. The thyroid is so powerful that its imbalance can cause a wide range of symptoms and problems including heart disease and heart failure. That said, doing all of the prior steps in this book will often cause your body to balance its hormones (it will heal itself). But, should you still feel especially bad, then I would suggest a visit to a doctor who specializes in this type of treatment.

If your doctor is not willing to test your hormones or run complete panels for which you ask, please seek out an FDN (Functional Diagnostic Nutrition) practitioner or go to the website, www.healthcheckusa.com and you can order these test right online and receive a full explanation of their labs as well.

In the 1950s, Dr. Broda Barnes conducted a study patterned after the famous Framingham study. The Framingham Study supposedly proved that a diet low in saturated fats reduces the risk of heart disease. In Framingham, 15% of residents were diagnosed with heart disease in spite of their "heart healthy" lifestyles. Residents were encouraged to stop smoking, lose weight, exercise and reduce their saturated fat intakes.

In the Barnes study (using a similar number of study paticipants, length of study, etc as Framingham), no one was asked to change their lifestyle, even if that meant to stop smoking. Barnes evaluated patients for hypothyroidism (low performing thyroid) based solely on symptoms, and, if present, treated them with Armour Thyroid (a natural thyroid replacement made from dessicated pig thyroid). Barnes' results were astonishing. Unlike Framingham where 15% had heart disease following a "heart healthy lifestyle" the Barnes study group found heart disease in only two-tenths of one percent of members. This is a rather strong argument that the principle cause of heart disease is untreated hypothyroidism rather than merely diet and exercise.

Regarding hormone therapy, I strongly recommend you read the books *Overcoming Thyroid Disorders* and *The Miracle of Natural Hormones* both by Dr. David Brownstein to fully understand the need to address these issues.

Basically, if your hormone levels are low, or even in the low-normal range, they should probably be brought up to the high-normal range, especially if you are suffering symptoms such as fatigue, tremors, low libido, brittle nails and so forth. Brownstein's books provide long lists of symptoms that can indicate the need for treatment and the need to treat these problems with natural, non-synthetic hormones.

When I was first diagnosed with heart failure and began searching for answers, I found that my thyroid T3 level was in the low normal range. I asked my cardiologist if it would be prudent to treat it so that it would rise to high normal. "Why," he said, "it's normal." "Yes," I replied, "But my health is not normal and you have no other answers for me except to suggest a heart transplant." I found a doctor willing to treat me with natural thyroid and that was very likely one of the principle elements that allowed my heart to heal.

Ask your doctor for a full panel of blood tests on all of your hormones. Regarding your thyroid, be sure to ask for T1, T2, T3, T4 and reverse T3 tests; otherwise, they are likely to run only T4/TSH tests. Ask to get a copy of the results of all tests and use these when reading Dr. Brownstein's books.

I ended up taking Armour Thyroid, testosterone, melatonin, DHEA and human growth hormone when working to heal my heart. I still take three of those five in my regular routine to stay healthy.

SUGGESTED RECIPES

<u>Tom's Sweet Texas Tea</u>

½ gallon filtered water
4 tea bags (preferable decaffeinated)
1/3 cup raw, organic honey

Preparation
Bring water to a boil. Turn off heat and add tea bags. Let steep until the water temperature is 118 degrees (F) or slightly lower. Remove tea bags and stir in honey until dissolved. Refrigerate and drink. Do not add the honey at higher heat levels because it will kill off the essential enzymes you want from the honey.

<u>Roasted Organic Chicken</u>

1 3-lb whole organic chicken, giblets removed
Raw sea salt and black pepper(optional) to taste
Onion powder to taste
1 stalk celery, leaves removed
4 to 6 ounces pasture butter

Preparation
Preheat oven to 350 degrees F.
Wash chicken under cold water and pat dry. Place in roasting pan and season generously inside and out with salt and pepper. Place 3 tablespoons of butter into the cavity. Rub the exterior skin with the remaining butter, placing between the skin and meat wherever possible. Chop celery into 3 or 4 pieces and place into the cavity.
Bake uncovered 1 hour and 15 minutes in oven to a minimum internal temperature of 180 degrees F. Remove from heat and baste with melted butter and drippings. Cover with foil and allow to rest about 30 minutes before serving.

Remove meat from the bones and reserve bones for the broth below.

Lemon Chicken

This is incredibly easy and deceptively delicious.

1	3lb	organic chicken, cut up
1/3		fresh organic lemon juice
2	tbs	extra virgin olive oil
2	cloves	garlic, minced
1	teas	dried oregano
		Organic sea Salt to taste

Freshly ground black pepper to taste (optional)

Preparation

Rinse and dry chicken pieces and arrange skin side down in a glass baking dish. Season chicken generously with organic sea salt and then with freshly ground pepper. Whisk together all other ingredients and pour over chicken. Let stand for one hour.

Preheat oven to 400 degrees F. Roast chicken in baking dish for 30 minutes. Turn the pieces skin side up and continue to roast until browned and juices run clear when a thigh is pierced, for about 30 to 45 minutes more. Remove from oven. Strain juices if desired and serve.

Bone Broth

1 large onion, quartered
1 large carrot, peeled and coarsely chopped
2 ribs celery coarsely chopped
4 cloves garlic, peeled
¼ cup raw, organic apple cider vinegar
Organic grass-fed beef bones (shanks are good) or Organic free-range chicken bones
Water

Preparation

If using chicken, break apart the carcass and place in the crock pot with all ingredients, covering with water. If using beef bones, I suggest first browning them in the oven. Place them on a non-aluminum cookie sheet or pan, drizzle a little extra virgin olive oil or coconut oil over the meat or bones and roast at 350 degrees F for about 35 minutes. If using shanks, remove the meat and save. Place bones in your crock pot and continue as with the chicken.

I usually set the crock pot on high for about one hour then turn to low for 24 to 48 hours. Strain the broth from the other ingredients. With the beef broth, I retrieve the meat and set it aside for the soup I will make later with the broth.

Fermented Vegetables

1 head organic green cabbage, thinly sliced and chopped
5 stalks organic celery, thinly sliced
2 garlic cloves, minced
2 to 3 tablespoons raw, organic sea salt
2 tablespoons whey (usually from my own yogurt)

Preparation

Place all ingredients, except the whey, in a large bowl, tossing the vegetables to spread the salt and let sit for one hour. Using clean hands, squish the vegetables forcing them to render their liquid.

Using a clean jar, begin transferring and packing down the vegetables into the jar. I use a small wooden "muddler" for the job. This will help extract even more of the juices. When the jar is full, add one to three tablespoon of whey (hopefully, you will be making your own yogurt as well, and you can use the whey floating at the top of the container), if you don't have whey, you can also use 2 or 3 tablespoons of the juice from a prior batch of fermented vegetables or from store bought sauerkraut such as Bubbies brand (which is naturally fermented).

Let the jars sit on the counter for one week, making sure that the liquid is higher than the top of the vegetable mixture. If necessary, place a small heavy object on the vegetables to keep them below the liquid line. Try to keep the room temperature between 70 and

80 degrees F. During the winter when my home is not in that temperature range, I often use the oven, door closed with the light on, as an alternate spot for the jar while the vegetables ferment. At the end of the week, refrigerate. Other vegetables I often add to this mixture are carrots, ginger, daikon, garlic, onions and often other root vegetables. Relax and be creative!!

Tom's Post-Workout Protein Shake

8 to 16 ounces	Homemade yogurt
One scoop	Whey protein powder
2 organic chickens	egg yolks, raw from organic, free-range
2 ounces	pomegranate juice

Mix together with a fork or spoon. Enjoy!

Tom's Nutrient-Dense "heal all" Southwest-Style Chicken Soup

2	tbs	Pasture Butter
1 ¼	lbs	Chopped or shredded cooked chicken
1	small	onion, chopped
2	ribs	celery, thinly sliced
1	small	red bell pepper, chopped
1 (optional)		jalapeno pepper, deseeded and chopped
3	cloves	garlic, minced
½	head	cabbage, shredded and chopped
2		zucchini, diced
3	cups	Chicken Bone Broth (homemade), or more if desired
2	teas	chili powder
1	teas	cumin
1	teas	Hungarian Paprika
¼	cup	dry white wine
1	teas	salt – or to taste

½	teas	pepper (optional)
1	15-oz can	pink or red beans
1	14-oz can	chopped tomatoes
2	tbls	tomato paste (optional)
		Cilantro, chopped (to taste)
		Sour cream
		Avocado

Preparation

Add butter to stock pot over medium high heat. Add chicken, onions, celery, garlic, bell pepper, jalapeno, cabbage and zucchini. Sauté until soft. Add stock and all seasonings, including cilantro. Add beans and tomatoes with liquid. Taste to adjust seasoning. Bring to a gentle boil and reduce heat to low. Simmer for about 20 minutes.

Serve with a dollop of sour cream and chopped avocado.

Granola

6	cups	oats
		Unsweetened coconut, to taste
		Pecans, to taste
		Walnuts, to taste
		Sunflower seeds, to taste
½	cup	coconut oil, warmed
½	cup	honey
¾	tsp	salt
1 ½	tsp	vanilla

Preparation

Soak oats for 24 hours in a combination of water with some yogurt and a little raw cider vinegar. Drain and rinse gently in wire mesh strainer
To the oats add the other dry ingredients.

Combine the coconut oil, honey, salt and vanilla and add to the oats mixture.

Spread mixture in a cookie sheet. Start drying mixture in a 200 degree oven and then reduce the heat to 170 degrees F. This process takes time, about 24 hours. Stir occasionally. Add dried fruit if you like. Store in a glass jar.

Apple Pie Oatmeal

This wonderful recipe is from Kelly the Kitchen Kop's website
2 ½	cups	organic oats (steel cut or regular, but I like regular best)
1	tbls	whole grain oat flour
1 ¾	cup	buttermilk (In place of buttermilk or yogurt or kefir for soaking, you can use 1 tablespoon of whey, lemon juice or vinegar to 1 cup of liquid, usually water for those who can't have dairy, but milk would be fine, too)
½	cup	organic coconut oil, melted
4		eggs
½	cup	real maple syrup or raw honey
1	teas	aluminum-free baking powder
½	teas	sea salt
2	tsp	cinnamon
2	tsp	vanilla
2	cups	raisins
2	cups	chopped apples, pear or other fruit of choice

Optional:
2	cups	chopped nuts

Preparation
Soak oats, flour and buttermilk covered on kitchen counter overnight, but 24 hours is better in order to break down more phytic acid. In the morning, beat oil, sugar, and eggs until glossy. Add baking powder, salt, cinnamon and vanilla; beat. Stir in oats, raisins, and chopped apples (or pears). You may need to add a little more milk at this point if the oats seem a little too dry. Pour into

9×13 buttered baking dish and bake at 350 for 20-40 minutes, depending on your desired consistency.

Serve with butter and a little more real maple syrup if desired, but it's really good all on its own!

One more thing: In case you're wondering why the oats don't need to be drained after soaking overnight, Jenny from Nourished Kitchen has this to say: "You don't have to because phytic acid is degraded. It doesn't leach into the water like oxalates."

Non-Fluoride Natural Tooth Powder[25]

½   cup   baking soda
10   drops   pure peppermint essential oil (this is not the same as peppermint extract or fragrance oil. Also, it should be a high quality food grade essential oil, which is available from many health food stores)
5   drops   myrrh essential oil (optional, also available in many health food stores)

Preparation
Mix all ingredients in a small jar with a lid, cover, and shake well to disperse the oils throughout. Use a small amount on a damp toothbrush the way you would use toothpaste.

The peppermint essential oil helps freshen breath, kill bacteria, and clear sinuses. The myrrh oil is highly antibacterial and anti-fungal It is often used in the ancient healing arts of Ayurvedic Medicine. The baking soda restores a natural, slightly alkaline pH balance to the teeth and gums and helps to whiten teeth.

REFERENCES & RESOURCES

Books

Nourishing Traditions by Sally Fallon
Statin Drugs, Side Effects and the Misguided War on Cholesterol by Duane Graveline, M.D.
Wheat Belly by William Davis, M.D.
Iodine: Why You Need It, Why You Can't Live Without It by David Brownstein, M.D.
Death By Modern Medicine by Caroline Dean, M.D. N.D.
The Magnesium Miracle by Caroline Dean, M.D. N.D.
Overcoming Thyroid Disorders by David Brownstein, M.D.
The Miracle of Natural Hormones by David Brownstein, M.D.
Drugs that Don't Work and Natural Therapies That Do! by David Brownstein, M.D.
Why Stomach Acid Is Good For You: Natural Relief from Heartburn, Indigestion, Reflux and GERD by Jonathan Wright
Radical Remission: Surviving Cancer Against All Odds by Kelly A. Turner Ph.D.
The Whole Soy Story by Kaayla Daniel, ph.D.
Hypothyroidism Type 2: The Epidemic by Mark Starr, M.D.
Minding My Mitochondria by Terry Wahls, M.D.
The Wahls Protocol by Terry Wahls, M.D.
The Omnivores Dilemma by Michael Pollan
Killing Cancer – Not People by Robert G. Wright
Alternative Medicine Definitive Guide to Cancer by W. John Diamond and W. Lee Cowden
Cure Tooth Decay: Heal and Prevent Cavities with Nutrition by Ramiel Nagel
Grain Brain by David Perlmutter, M.D.
Know Your Fats: The Complete Primer for Understanding the Nutrition of Fats, Oils and Cholesterol by Mary Enig
Breaking the Vicious Cycle by Elaine Gloria Gottschall
The Untold Story of Milk: The History, Politics and Science of Nature's Perfect Food by Ron Schmid

Malignant Medical Myths: Why Medical Treatment Causes 200,000 Deaths in the USA each Year and How to Protect Yourself by Joel Kaufman PhD
Heart Disease: What Your Doctor Won't Tell You by Rodger Murphree, M.D.
Salt Your Way To Health by David Brownstein, M.D.
Solved: The Riddle of Heart Attacks by Broda Barnes, M.D.
Good Calories. Bad Calories by Gary Taubes
Hypothyroidism, Health & Happiness: The Riddle of Illness Revealed by Steven F. Hotze, M.D.
Food is Your Best Medicine by Henry G. Bieler, M.D.
Vitamin B-12 for Health by Dr. David Brownstein, M.D.
Eat Fat. Lose Fat by Mary Enig
The Paleo Manifesto: Ancient Wisdom for Lifelong Health by John Durant
Fermented by Jill Ciciarelli.
How Doctors Think by Jerome Groopman, M.D.
The Cure For Heart Disease: Truth Will Save A Nation by Dwight Lundell, M.D.

Online Resources

Weston A. Price Foundation: www.westonaprice.org
Center for Holistic Medicine: www.drbrownstein.com
Life Extension Foundation: www.lef.org
A Wise Approach: awiseapproach.wordpress.com
Broda Barnes Foundation: www.brodabarnes.org
Food Matters: www.foodmatters.tv
One Percent Health: www.OnePercentHealth.com
Empowered Sustenance: www.EmpoweredSustenance.com
Whitaker Wellness Institute: www.whitakerwellness.com
Dr. Dean Silver: http://deansilvermd.com
Dr. Terry Wahls: www.TerryWahls.com
Dr. Julia Schulenburg: www.holistichealingjs.com
For a Functional Diagnostic Nutritionist:
www.healthcheckusa.com
Farrar Family Chiropractic: http://www.farrarchiro.com/

Kelly the Kitchen Kop: www.kellythekitchenkop.com
www.facebook.com/KellytheKitchenKop
Ancient Minerals: http://www.ancient-minerals.com/
Primal Pit Paste: http://www.primalpitpaste.com/
Bio-Kult: http://www.bio-kult.com/
Eden Foods: http://www.edenfoods.com/
Bubbies Foods: http://www.bubbies.com/
Rapunzel Foods: http://www.rapunzel.de/uk/p_suessung.html
The Gerson Institute: http://gerson.org/gerpress/
Camelot Cancer Care: http://www.camelotcancercare.com/
Kangen Water Systems: http://www.enagic.com/
Synergy Kombucha: http://www.synergydrinks.com/
Bragg Foods: http://www.bragg.com/

Recommended movies and documentaries

...first, do no harm
Lorenzo's Oil
Food Matters
Fat, Sick and Nearly Dead
Fat Head
The Gerson Miracle
A Beautiful Truth
Burzinski Parts I and II
King Corn
Hungry for Change

References

1   http://www.huffingtonpost.com/dana-ullman/homeopathic-medicine-_b_1258607.html

2   http://articles.mercola.com/sites/articles/archive/2003/11/26/death-by-medicine-part-one.aspx

3   http://www.undergroundhealth.com/symptoms-of-aspartame-poisoning/

4   http://articles.mercola.com/sites/articles/archive/2009/10/13
     /artificial-sweeteners-more-dangerous-than-you-ever-
     imagined.aspx

5   http://www.motherearthnews.com/natural-health/gmo-safety-
     zmgz13amzsto.aspx

6   https://www.facebook.com/photo.php?v=101537675847555
     00
     https://www.facebook.com/photo.php?v=101537675847555
     0

7   http://onepercenthealth.blogspot.com/2013/06/twelve-
     reasons-to-cut-canola-oil.html

8   http://onepercenthealth.blogspot.com/2013/02/coconut-oil-
     reverses-amyotrphiic.html

9   http://www.beliefnet.com/columnists/watchwomanonthewal
     l/2013/01/alzheimers-doctors-taking-note-of-coconut-oil-
     helps-aspergers-autistism-parkinsons-als-dementia-
     multiple-sclerosis-diabetes.html

10   http://articles.mercola.com/sites/articles/archive/2010/05/18
     /microwave-hazards.aspx

11   http://truthstreammedia.com/epa-to-raise-allowable-
     glyphosate-levels-in-food-crops-3000/

12   http://onepercenthealth.blogspot.com/2014/01/yogurt-
     spoonful-of-powerful-nutritional.html

13   http://www.healthytheory.com/corn-fed-vs-grass-fed-beef

14   http://blog.lef.org/2012/09/organic-foods-are-better-for-
     you.html?utm_source=facebook&utm_medium=social&ut
     m_campaign=normal

15 *Journal of Applied Ecology*, Volume 50, Issue 4, pages 851-862

16 http://kellythekitchenkop.com/2008/08/healthy-fats-oils.html

17 http://www.lef.org/vitamins-supplements/item01814/Two-Per-Day-Capsules.html?source=search&key=twoperday%20capsules

18 http://onepercenthealth.blogspot.com/2013/07/the-remarkable-anticancer-properties-of.html

19 http://www.sciencedirect.com/science/article/pii/S073510978680 2935

20 http://onepercenthealth.blogspot.com/2013/03/coq10-and-cancer-treatment.html

21 http://www.westonaprice.org/childrens-health/vaccinations-parents-informed-choice

22 http://www.ibtimes.co.uk/brain-damaged-uk-victims-swine-flu-vaccine-get-60-million-compensation-1438572#.UxO516V3xpg.wordpress

23 http://www.consumerreports.org/cro/magazine-archive/2011/january/food/mercury-in-tuna/overview/index.htm

24 http://www.ewg.org/research/healthy-home-tips/tip-6-skip-non-stick-avoid-dangers-teflon

25 http://foodmatters.tv/articles-1/make-your-own-natural-toothpaste

26 http://onepercenthealth.blogspot.com/2013/01/the-benefits-of-high-cholesterol-by.html

27 http://onepercenthealth.blogspot.com/2013/02/artificial-sweetners-fda-approved.html

28   http://vactruth.com/2009/12/14/mercury-in-flu-vaccine-is-250-times-higher-than-classified-hazardous-waste/

29   http://antivaccine.wordpress.com/2013/10/24/facts-regarding-the-misleading-claim-that-mercury-thimerosal-has-been-removed-from-vaccines/

30   http://www.doctoroz.com/videos/dr-joel-fuhrmans-nutrition-density-chart

31   http://www.raw-wisdom.com/coffee-enemas

32   http://onepercenthealth.blogspot.com/2013/12/surprising-effect-of-probiotics-outside.html

33   Chapter 6, Antacids in *Drugs that Don't Work and Natural Therapies That Do!* by Dr. David Brownstein

34   http://blog.drbrownstein.com/statins-increase-breast-cancer-by-over-200/

35   http://www.foodmatters.tv/articles-1/oil-pulling-the-habit-that-can-transform-your-health

36   *Malignant Medical Myths* by Joel Kaufman Pages 259-277

37   http://articles.mercola.com/sites/articles/archive/2014/03/25/philippines-dental-amalgam.aspx

38   http://articles.mercola.com/sites/articles/archive/2014/03/22/aluminum-toxicity-alzheimers.aspx

39   http://www.realfoodnutrients.com/NewsletterArticles/SomethingYouveNeverBeenToldAboutBreakfastCereals.htm

40   http://donoteatthis.com/2010/12/27/mcdonalds-chicken-mcnuggets-made-of-corn-and-chemicals/

41   http://articles.mercola.com/sites/articles/archive/2013/03/13/unlabeled-aspartame-use.aspx

42   http://onepercenthealth.blogspot.com/2013/01/the-amazing-dr-terry-wahl-there-are.html

43   http://www.thehealthyhomeeconomist.com/aspartame-with-milk-may-trigger-brain-seizures/#more-11269

CPSIA information can be obtained
at www.ICGtesting.com
Printed in the USA
FFOW03n1317290117
31771FF